PRAISE FOR LONG LIVE THE QUEEN

"This book could not be more timely. As our world seems to be falling apart around us, demanding sacrifice, self-control and the courage to carry on, Bryan Kozlowski presents us with the salutary example of a woman who has lived a life of purpose and discipline in the service of something greater than herself. Thoroughly conversant with the serious and popular literature on the Queen, and much else besides, he writes in a style so engaging and fun that one might miss his very serious and useful message for our times."

—Robert Bucholz, professor of history, Loyola University, Chicago

"*Long Live the Queen!* made me feel like I was eavesdropping on Oscar Wilde, the Queen Mum, and Malcolm Gladwell at one of Her Majesty's garden parties. Witty, charming, historically astute, often wickedly funny and always genuinely inspiring, Bryan Kozlowski surprises readers on every page with adroit insight into Queen Elizabeth II's life and practical applications for royal improvements to our own. Whether you're an ingenue intrigued by The Crown or a lifelong loyal subject of the sovereign, *Long Live the Queen!* is a must-read."

—Dudley Delffs, author of *The Faith of Queen Elizabeth*

"With reverence and humor, Bryan Kozlowski has written an intriguing rationale for why Queen Elizabeth is so long-lived. Part biography, part self-help, this look at Her Majesty through 23 Rules for Living is a fun—and instructional—read for a wider audience than just royal watchers."

—Anne Easter Smith, author of *A Rose for the Crown, Queen by Right,* and *This Son of York*

"With Queen Elizabeth II securing her status as longest-reigning monarch in the world, Bryan Kozlowski's book comes at an opportune moment. Equally entertaining and erudite, *Long Live the Queen!* explores what keeps this 94-year-old going. Her rules, it turns out, might well just apply to all of us."

—Arianne Chernock, associate professor of history, Boston University

"Scientifically fascinating, beautifully written and immensely practical, Kozlowski's compelling narrative is a book I recommend to all my patients. His meticulous research has unveiled the 23 most important steps to vibrant health and lasting vitality—presented as a thrilling page-turner."

—Dr. Helena Popovic, author of *NeuroSlimming: Let Your Brain Change Your Body*

"Engaging, insightful, and wonderfully grounding at a time when the world needs it most. *Long Live the Queen* allows readers a thoroughly enjoyable peek inside the life of the most famous woman on Earth and lets us in on the secrets to her tremendous health and success for over nine decades....From page one, Kozlowski's words had me believing that a brighter, more serene future lies ahead. It's not her servants or her position that make Queen Elizabeth's life remarkable—it's the simplicity and sense of purpose with which she lives each day. I intend to read this book several times in the coming years as a touchstone in my personal quest for a calm yet more productive life."

—Melanie Summers, author of *The Royal Treatment*

"As someone who has specialized in Queen Elizabeth I, I found *Long Live the Queen!*, about the second Queen Elizabeth a great pleasure to read. The author offers advice on how to eat, play, work, love, and possibly the most useful, age like a queen...This is a book to delight all who are interested in the monarchy."

—Carole Levin, professor of history, University of Nebraska, author of *The Heart and Stomach of a King*

"In depth research combined with expert commentary and humor gives insight into the Queen's character and royal rituals, helping explain just why she has ruled so long."

—Becky Libourel Diamond, research historian, author of *The Thousand Dollar Dinner*

"Entertaining and insightful...an engaging royal guide to life!"

—Dr. Carolyn Harris, author of *Raising Royalty: 1000 Years of Royal Parenting*

Long Live
the Queen!

Turner Publishing Company
Nashville, Tennessee
www.turnerpublishing.com

Cover design: Lauren Peters-Collaer
Text design and composition by Karen Sheets de Gracia in the Palace Script, Mrs Eaves, and Adobe Garamond typefaces.

Library of Congress Cataloging-in-Publication Data Upon Request

Printed in the United States of America

20 21 22 23 24   10 9 8 7 6 5 4 3 2 1

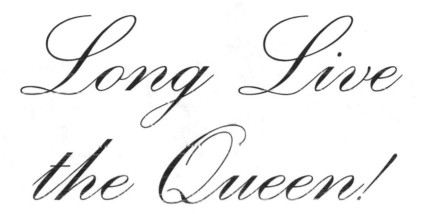

Long Live the Queen!

23 RULES FOR LIVING

FROM BRITAIN'S LONGEST-REIGNING MONARCH

Bryan Kozlowski

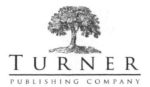

TURNER
PUBLISHING COMPANY

For Kristin, the loveliest sister in the land.

What do you mean by "If you really are a Queen"?
What right have you to call yourself so?
You ca'n't be a Queen, you know, till
you've passed the proper examination.
And the sooner we begin it, the better.

—Lewis Carroll, *Through the Looking Glass*

Contents

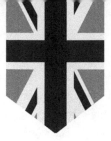

GOD SAVE MY GRACIOUS ME

OR, THE WHITE MAGIC OF WINDSOR

As far as I can see, some people have to be
fed royalty like sea-lions fish.
—LADY STRATHMORE, MATERNAL GRANDMOTHER OF ELIZABETH II

It's a curious sensation, to those who have felt it. So very much like a "high," one is tempted to begin with a drug-related analogy (though I'm wary of mixing up narcotics with Her Majesty's good name). And what would be an appropriate royal parallel? It feels like a drop of ecstasy in a bracing cup of Earl Grey? I didn't think to record the particulars the first time I experienced it, or imagine how much it would change the way I live. The whole thing began so inauspiciously. Come to think of it, it caught me as unaware as most mind altering highs usually catch out naive new initiates—half asleep and in my pajamas.

I remember it was early, *very* early, on the morning of April 29, 2011, otherwise known as the wedding day of Prince William and Catherine Middleton. Feeling like a groggy version of Ethelred the Unready, I wasn't quite sure what I was doing up at this hour, stumbling in the dark to turn on the television, momentarily blinded by the frenzied mass of waving Union Jacks. It certainly wasn't due to any obsession with the royal family whom, at the moment, I was finding slightly hard to forgive for arranging the whole "wedding of the century" thing in the morning, without apparent thought for the inconvenience posed on their ex-colonists across the pond. At the time, I was no more intrigued by the workings of royalty than a rush-hour commuter is intrigued by the occasional glimpse of a rainbow across the freeway. It was pretty when it popped out from its lofty abode, and I was content to simply stare. To watch the pageantry of a royal wedding, to be just another spectator of this ancient, beautiful and, perhaps, rather silly spectacle was good enough for me. And when all the hoohah was over, to promptly stumble back to bed was my only ambition. I was *not* one of Lady Strathmore's sea-lions barking for more. Or so I thought. But oh no; this royal rainbow had its way with me.

As the dawn rose and the Abbey choirboys sang and the trumpets blared and the sea of fascinators bobbed merrily in their pews, some sort of strange magic took over. If I may briefly sound like a spacey druid, that morning Westminster Abbey felt like a power outlet, pulsating sheer joy, the heart of euphoria on earth, and I was plugged in, baby! I felt more alive, more human, more capable of checking off whatever to-do list I could possibly dream up. I might even have attempted a semi-successful cartwheel to mark the occasion, something which normally filled me with bodily dread. But I didn't analyze the experience or chalk it up to anything more than simply the thrill of watching a live television event (with the cross-reference thought that, yes, perhaps I needed to get out more).

The encounter would have passed me by entirely if it wasn't for the premier, years later, of a little show on Netflix called *The Crown*. Watching it brought back something similar to what I experienced on Will and Kate's wedding day—an irresistible urge for personal improvement. There was something contagious in the way actress Claire Foy portrayed Elizabeth Windsor. Episode one had hardly finished and I was already standing taller and conducting myself with more bodily grace and decorum. I stopped short at trying to learn the Queen's cut-glass accent (I totally didn't), but you get the picture. Apparently watching the splendor of monarchy—even via a dramatized miniseries—brought out the better, more polished side of me. I reckoned there were only two possible explanations: either I'm a long-lost royal simply acting out my natural destiny (I'd settle for Anastasia's fourteenth cousin) or I'm just a royal dweeb.

＊

Turns out it was nothing so personal. With the hindsight of an entire book behind me, I can now say that I was simply an unconscious participant in a universal phenomenon affecting millions throughout history. Its roots lay in a fascinating blend of cultural anthropology, quasi-religious symbolism and tribal magic. The ancient Greeks had a closely related word for the concept—*kalokagathia*, an ideal of personal grace and beauty, believed to be the birthright of the high born, which often inspired yearnings of excellence in lesser mortals. Watching the great and good stirs us to greater goodness. In other words, royalty tends to rub off on its spectators. And rather fantastically, the British monarchy is one of the last remaining institutions where you can still observe and experience *kalokagathia*, in its purest form, today.

Royal researcher Jeremy Paxman calls it the "benign influence" of the Crown, something that makes countless cynics drop a curtsey in front of the Queen and impels many more to stand bolt upright in their living rooms, should Her Majesty appear on their television sets. Helen Mirren famously experienced the sensation during her Oscar-winning performance in the film *The Queen*. Brought up with staunch anti-monarchist tendencies, Mirren admitted to previously having "a Sex Pistols attitude to the Royal Family," explaining, "It wasn't a world I was enamoured with." Yet her on-screen role as Elizabeth II worked an inward alchemy, gradually transforming Mirren into a self-proclaimed "Queenist" who felt no shame in shouting Elizabeth's praises to a bunch of equally bemused Americans on Oscar night. "I basically fell in love with [her]," said Mirren.

Loyalists and scoffers alike have tried for decades to winkle out how and why this all works so successfully, how the Crown—currently occupied by an unassuming grandmother, barely over five feet tall, with absolutely no political power—can exert such tremendous power where it counts most. Though most agree the mystery lies in the fact that the British Crown is ultimately reflective and, for an unelected institution, far more representative than you might think. As writer Rebecca West once famously opined, to look upon the splendor of monarchy is to see "magnified images of ourselves . . . but better, ourselves behaving well." A sentiment earlier echoed by *The Times* of 1936: "The Queen has come to be the symbol of every side of life of this society, its universal representative in whom her people see their better selves ideally reflected." For Robert Lacey, royal historian for *The Crown*, kingship gives us a peek into "the majesty of the ordinary man."*

People once shamelessly spoke of the English aristocracy as "our betters" for a similar reason—in them they saw a more polished reflection of themselves. Class systems have evolved, no doubt, but the impulse appears ingrained. For instance, it usually stuns the press that crime rates tend to go *down* during big royal events. Newspapers in London once braced for a dramatic surge in thefts on Elizabeth's coronation day in 1953. Nobody knew what a tightly packed mob of 30,000 onlookers could get up to. Their best behavior, so it seemed. There was a surprising *decrease* in thefts that day. It happened again in the 1980s. Despite one of the biggest precautionary police forces deployed for Prince Charles and Diana's wedding, nothing unorderly took place. "There is something about a royal show which mysteriously reduces the crime rate on the day to negligible figures instead of quadrupling it as everyone expects," writes biographer Elizabeth Longford, who attributes "the common source of grace" to "royalty itself." A grace which extends to children too.

When researchers asked a group of young schoolboys in London what they would do if the Queen dropped by for a visit, one Paul Pitchely imagined big improvements at home. He would make his bed, sweep the floors, paint the house, do the dishes and, just to be sure, "I would put some money in the meater so the lights would not go off half frow [sic] the dinner . . ." Only the language of fairy tales seems appropriate for such a motivating influence for good. To one observant housewife, who felt all the royal tingles on coronation day 1953, it was just that. Nothing less than "White Magic," she said, was behind it all.

Royalty's ability to cast this spell over the public, to *literally* make people better, has deep roots in English history. For hundreds of years faithful British subjects gathered in droves outside Westminster, anxious to receive the "royal touch"—a conviction that one caress of

---

* Which further explains why it is so oddly discombobulating when even minor royals misbehave. Logically we shouldn't care, but we do because they are ultimately symbols of us. "When some of them did badly, we did not like what we saw of ourselves," says historian William Shawcross.

the monarch's hand would cure them of certain disfiguring diseases.* Elizabeth's seventeenth-century predecessor, Charles II, was such an indefatigable touching machine, he laid hands on more than 90,000 people during his reign. Naturally, to perform this and other duties for the country, the health of the monarch had to be preserved. So it wasn't long before, in the public's imagination, the King or Queen's health was symbolically linked to the health of the nation itself, a legacy still strongly with us. Consider England's unofficial national anthem. The "save" in "God Save the Queen" derives from *salvus*, Latin for "healthy," making the anthem a veritable plea to keep the monarch fighting fit, and likewise the country as a whole.

This symbiotic relationship is most evident on days of national rejoicing. Whenever the English have something grandiose to celebrate, they naturally congregate—not outside government buildings or the prime minister's residence but the monarch's official home, Buckingham Palace. As Winston Churchill once observed, "a great battle is lost: parliament turns out the government. A great battle is won: crowds cheer the Queen." Evidently the modern psyche still requires a *kalokagathia*, someone to act out the grace and greatness we wish to see in ourselves.

*

Arguably no other monarch in British history has understood that role or performed it more successfully than Elizabeth II. For nearly 70 years on the throne, she has never wavered in her belief in what *The Times* said of her back in 1953: "In her is incarnate . . . the whole of society. . . . She represents the life of her people." To preserve her own life to the best of her ability is nothing less than her constitutional duty. So much of the Queen's daily routine is fueled by this royal drive for survival, even down to the way she shakes people's hands and the temperature of her afternoon tea. Elizabeth is "singularly blessed," says biographer Craig

---

* Readers of *The Lord of the Rings* may recognize this as the historical inspiration behind the healing powers of Tolkien's hero king, Aragorn. Through curing Faramir, Éowyn and Merry in the Houses of Healing, he is recognized as the rightful ruler of Gondor, fulfilling the prophecy that "the hands of a king are the hands of a healer."

Brown, "with what Evelyn Waugh once called the 'the sly, sharp instinct for self-preservation.'" To test the strength of that instinct is only to look at her ongoing achievements in longevity. In 2015 Elizabeth broke the monarchial record, surpassing her great-great-grandmother Queen Victoria as Britain's longest-reigning sovereign. She's currently on her *fourteenth* prime minister (matching George III's hitherto unmatchable record) and has indirectly given Prince Charles his own less flattering claim to fame: Charles has now waited longer to assume the throne than any heir in English history.

Yet unlike other modern royals, Elizabeth has never needed a "life-style manager" or health coach or personal trainer or therapist to achieve these record feats. By her own assessment, she was simply "trained" for the task from childhood. "You can do a lot if you're properly trained," she once told a soldier she was commending for bravery, "and I hope I have been." The Queen underwent the core of this training during a specific era in Britain and within a certain societal framework prac-tically unrecognizable today—a generation that approached living, working, eating and emoting very differently from us. To playwright Alan Bennett, Elizabeth is "a living archive" of a rapidly fading past, one of the last stalwart icons of a generation that tackled life—its struggles and joys—with far more pluck and good sense. Like the Star of the Order's motto, emblazoned on the blue satin cape she wears on special occasions, the Queen herself is a true *Auspicium Melioris Aevi*, a "token of a better age."

Even her critics can't ignore her accumulated wisdom. Writing on the milestone of the Queen's eightieth birthday, the *Guardian* (hardly a loyalist newspaper) had to concede the utterly remarkable: "She has served in a demanding role, that of head of state, for half a century and has made barely a mistake. . . . By the usual measures—namely sustained popularity and an ability to avoid trouble—Elizabeth Windsor would have to be judged one of the most accomplished politicians of the modern era, albeit as a non-politician." Little wonder Prince William looks more and more to the Queen these days for inspiration. In prepa-ration for his own role as future King, he once jokingly admitted to longing for a sort of pocket-size reference guide to his grandmother's extraordinary life, to, as he says, "take all of her experiences, all of her knowledge and put it in a small box and be able to constantly refer to it."

✳

In a modest way, I like to think of this book as that "small box"—an owner's manual to upgrading to QE2.0 for yourself. In it we'll explore the habits, coping techniques and traditions Elizabeth has embraced over her long reign, how she differs from other royals—past and present— and how her life's work has extended her lifespan itself. Essentially, we'll examine the inner workings of "Queendom" (if I may be allowed to quote the honorable Queen Latifah). And since Buckingham Palace is a stickler for order, you'll find the material brewed down into a collection of tidy rules. I rather naturally arrived at 23 of them; no doubt others could come up with many more. Twenty-three, however, felt like an appropriate numerical celebration. It was on April 23, 2019, that Elizabeth officially became not only the longest-reigning British monarch, but also the longest-*living* monarch in the world.

More importantly, these 23 rules are designed not just to be theoretically admired from a distance but to be followed on a daily basis (be you knighted a Sir, Dame or among the rankless hoi polloi like myself). To be a role model is what the Queen is there for, after all. As Elizabeth's first Archbishop of Canterbury put it, the Queen was specially anointed to lead her people "in the way wherein they should go." To inspire us to act a little more *queenish* is part of her royal duty. We are, I now proudly admit it, sea-lions in need of some royal fish. And Elizabeth has a lifetime's bucketful.

Though a quick note to clarify . . .

Acting more like thelatest-and-greatest in a long line of British monarchsdoesn't mean going all regal and imperious. If you're starting to dazzle your friends and family with impersonations of Elizabeth Taylor playing Cleopatra—"You will therefore assume the position of a suppliant before this throne. You will kneel."—I'm afraid you've started off on the wrong foot. Because paradoxically, to go to the tippy top of the social ladder, to mimic the ways and means of someone who has always lived with either "Highness" or "Majesty" in their title, is to step into the shoes of one of the most sensible and down-to-earth humans alive. Helen Mirren, who literally spent months acting like the Queen, confirms the experience in her autobiography, *In the Frame*:

> Out of nowhere, or maybe out of the hours of watching tape, or simply
> out of the effect the clothes had on me, I slipped into [Elizabeth's] walk
> and into her head and found it to be the most comfortable place to be. . . .
> From then on, I loved wearing those clothes and shoes, loved being that
> character that I thought of as the captain of a submarine, deep and in
> control, but with a kind of simplicity. . . . I don't think I have ever felt so
> comfortable playing a character as I did with Elizabeth II.

It might be difficult to imagine how monarchy can become so
deeply personal and transformative. But whether you call it "benign
influence" or "White Magic," the Queen herself has long recognized
the reality of the connection we all can potentially share with her. "I
want to show that the Crown is not merely an abstract symbol of our
unity," said Elizabeth in her first Christmas broadcast, "but a personal
and living bond between you and me." Feeling the spark of that connection years ago, watching a royal wedding in my pj's, I can't help but be
drawn to the deeper resonance of one of my all-time favorite Palace
stories. Years back, a simple exchange between Elizabeth's father, George
VI, and Princess Margaret prompted the younger to ask a wonderfully
perceptive question of the King. "Papa," she asked, "[when you sing the
royal anthem], do you sing, 'God Save My Gracious Me'?" The King
burst out laughing, but he remembered the episode his entire life.

The living bond between us and the Crown invites you and me
to ask the same glorious question, to sing ourselves into the same royal
hymnbook. Elizabeth has led the way for nearly seven decades, treating
her body and mind—for her country, her people and her ancient family—
as reverently as a Crown Jewel. Now it's your turn to learn a rule or two (or
23) from her brilliant life, to unleash your inner Westminster choirboy
and bellow out a lifelong chorus of "God Save My Gracious Me."*

---

* Or for the less regally minded, the humbler words of Roald Dahl's Big Friendly Giant work
just as well, for starters: "We is off! . . . We is off to meet Her Majester the Queen!"

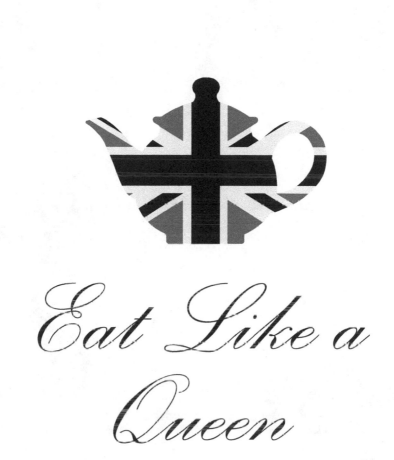

Eat Like a Queen

Sometimes it is worth explaining that we put it on specially;
we do not actually live like this all the time.

—ELIZABETH II ON EATING OFF GOLD PLATES, RESERVED FOR STATE BANQUETS

"**Y**ou will *not* photograph the Queen eating or drinking." It's one of the first injunctions photographers hear upon entering the Palace. Apparently it smacks too much of prerevolutionary France. Going all googly-eyed at the prospect of simply *watching* the monarch eat rarely caught on in England. After beheading Charles I, the English seem to have gradually lost their appetite for such courtly frippery. But not entirely. In fact, anyone invited to dine at Buckingham Palace today can still find traces of such royal-watching in action. And no matter what the photographers are told, to ensure a pleasant meal at the Palace, it's always advisable to keep a watchful eye on the Queen.

The solemn rites of royal etiquette still mean Elizabeth reigns supreme at the table. It might be one of her lesser-known prerogatives, but the Queen can ultimately determine how much (or how little) her guests eat by deciding, at any moment, to put her knife and fork down. And once she does, her staff gear into action, clearing everyone's plate, regardless of whether they have finished or not. Queen Victoria was an infamous, if somewhat tyrannical, upholder of the custom, and Elizabeth's father insisted on keeping up the tradition well into the twentieth century. No one received a second helping if the King didn't fancy one himself.

While Elizabeth has relaxed the practice over the years, it still underpins the running of her State Banquets. As former royal chef Darren McGrady explains, once the Queen puts down her cutlery, an ever-watchful page behind her presses a button on a handheld zapper, which sends a literal green-light signal to the kitchen, ushering in the next course. "Even if you are not finished, the course is over," said McGrady. Consequently, for Palace courtiers in the know (and those who wish to hang on to their beef Wellingtons), slyly watching the Queen and eating by her example is just smart dining. To use an expression from the world of scientific research, Elizabeth is a true "pacesetter," someone who influences how those around her eat.

Pacesetters, of course, aren't unique to the Palace; they abound in everyday life. They are the people—family members, coworkers, friends—who unconsciously motivate or tempt you to mimic their eating habits. They're the ones who influence you to order a side salad at a restaurant or a large order of fries instead, which is why pacesetters should always be chosen wisely. And personally, I can't think of any eater more worthy of mimicking than the Queen.

Here is a woman who has spent her life surrounded by the same food temptations that destroyed the health of many of her predecessors, yet she tackles the bounty with a seemingly endless spring of willpower. Guests who visit her at Balmoral say the place is so overrun with food temptations, "if you indulged thoroughly," observed Tony Blair, you could "put on a stone in a weekend." The Queen, on the other hand, has basically remained the same petite size over the years. She lived through a war which instilled her with unemotional attitudes towards her next meal, yet she would never dream of living without the daily treats she's come to love. In short, the Queen's table epitomizes the dieter's dream, what journalist Rachel Cooke calls "the strange coupling of decadence and moderation" which "pretty much sums up the royal family's attitude to food."

To be sure, the coupling presents a conundrum to those who think about food in the usual dieting sense, and buckets of ink have been spilled trying to understand her royal secret. But if there *is* a secret, it isn't in a special food plan (like her long-lived mother, the Queen has never been interested in dieting) but in a series of small strategies that have made a big impact over her lifetime. "Food is such an important start to sane thinking," observed the Queen Mother, who lived to be 101. On busy days meeting foreign dignitaries or keeping the Commonwealth together, food might be one of the least things on Elizabeth's mind, but her engine of monarchy is undoubtedly fueled by the unique way she thinks about it. Beginning with . . .

THE TUPPERWARE LADY
OR RULE #1—DON'T BE A
DRAMA-FOOD-QUEEN

Middle-class "foodies" are often no more enlightened than the rest of us. . . .
Their patronising and sneering sometimes makes one long for the old,
pre-foodie-revolution days, when the higher classes considered it vulgar to
make any comment at all on the food they were served.

—KATE FOX, *WATCHING THE ENGLISH*

The story *could* have been explosive. In 2003 a lone reporter from the *Daily Mirror* had infiltrated the heart of Buckingham Palace. Posing as an ordinary footman, he roamed the corridors incognito, eavesdropping on royal conversations and snapping pictures inside the most famous private home on the planet. It was a stakeout any paparazzo would give his telescoping front teeth for. So you can imagine the surprise when the less-than–Pulitzer Prize-winning headlines started surfacing. Forget the obvious scandal—the massive breach in Palace security—the most memorable jaw-dropper of the entire exposé was a bit more, well, domestic. According to the furtive footman, who produced a grainy photograph as proof, the Queen's breakfast cereals are brought to her table not in fine china or sparkling crystal but in (now prepare yourself for the bombshell) plastic *Tupperware* containers.

It was official: the press's infatuation with royal trivia had soared to goofy heights. But for all its absurdity, and despite the honest efforts of

Palace staff members to set the record straight (Her Majesty would never be served from anything which boasted a "burping seal," thank you very much), the story stuck in the public's imagination—not so much from shock than from a kind of cozy reassurance. After all, most of her subjects haven't seen the Queen change her hairdo in over 70 years, they know she *likes* wearing sensible shoes and unfashionable scarves and have grown up with the rumor that she goes around the Palace turning off lights to save energy. Spooning her morning cereal from a cheap, resealable container just seemed like something the Queen would naturally do: that when it came to food, she would be her usual, magnificently unfussy self. They were absolutely correct.

Straightforward simplicity has marked the Queen's dining habits since childhood. "She is not particular about food," a Palace official told biographer Sally Bedell Smith. "To her food is just fuel." An attitude which has had ironic ramifications on Palace life, especially when the Queen sits down to meals which are often less elaborate than her servants'. During the early years of their marriage, for instance, Elizabeth and Philip would contently dine on something simple: cold meat and salad or sausage with mashed potatoes. But this almost plebeian fare hardly passed muster downstairs. As one footman at the time remembers, "That sort of meal might be all right for the Royals, but it wasn't good enough for the staff," who felt their rights infringed upon if they didn't sit down to a three-course dinner or "high tea." Their boss, however, simply isn't interested in tickling her tongue with new flavor experiences, something her personal chefs quickly discover. Darren McGrady, who cooked for the royal family for years, recounts how he once sent a menu suggestion to the Queen for a snazzy new dish called Veiled Farmer's Daughter. "She sent a note back," recalls McGrady, "saying who or what are the 'Veiled Farmer's Daughter'?"

Needless to say, politicians who visit the Queen at Balmoral, priming their taste buds for a Michelin-star experience, are in for a shock. They arrive "expecting banquets," says journalist Jeremy Paxman, but instead get "an endless series of barbecues, with Prince Philip grilling the chops and sausages." For those demanding a bigger culinary show, the royal family have long been considered *a bit naff* (Brit slang for "comically lacking in style"). Indeed when the president of China visited London in 2005, he outright refused to stay at Buckingham Palace, citing it was "not five-star enough." The Queen is said to have the perfect comeback for all such pampered toffs. Replying to a guest complaining about the food at one of her State Banquets, she couldn't help but observe that "people don't come here because of the food; they come to eat off gold plates."

This pragmatism has doubtless made Elizabeth immensely easy to cook for over the years. "Cooking for [her] is no trouble at all," concluded Charles Mellis, after a twelve-year stint in the royal kitchens. Most of his colleagues would agree, breathing daily sighs of relief for the Queen's undemanding appetite and few legitimate dislikes.* There are occasions, of course, when the Queen is not entirely amused by her dinner, and for such times, there exists a notepad near her table for the express purpose of jotting down helpful hints to the kitchen. But complaining about food runs so contrary to her nature, she rarely uses it. There was the odd moment, years ago, when a footman found a torn off page from the notepad, concealing a squashed slug inside. "I found this in my salad," the Queen had scribbled on the pad. "Could you eat it?" Otherwise, as long as grubs stay out of her greens, the pad typically remains blank.

✳

None of this would be unusual if Elizabeth was simply a village granny with unstuffy tastes, but as head of the House of Windsor, she is a fascinating anomaly. For as historians are well aware, Elizabeth comes from

---

* There are only a handful of royal food no-no's, though most have a logical basis in either self-preservation or diplomacy. The Queen will not eat shellfish when traveling abroad, to avoid the risk of food poisoning, and won't touch anything infused with garlic, because no one likes a whiffy Queen. Further specifics about Elizabeth's genuine likes and dislikes have been purposefully kept to a minimum. She will never, for instance, "share" a picture of her prandial adventures on social media. She wouldn't understand why anyone would seriously care, for one, and wouldn't want to invite needless criticism, for another. "I have no intention of telling people what I have for breakfast," as Princess Margaret was wont to say. To appreciate the wisdom, I refer you to Meghan Markle's unfortunate episode with a posted image of avocado toast in 2019.

a long line of what the Queen Mother would call "complicated eaters." Her family tree is a veritable smorgasbord of royal foodies. Distant uncle Henry VIII famously stuffed himself to a 54-inch waist. George I and II were infamous overindulgers. Queen Victoria had such a weakness for sweets, she became little more than "a big round ball on wobbly legs" to her relations. King Edward VII—nicknamed "Tum-Tum"—practically demanded his guests keep pace with his gargantuan feeding habits. Near the front door of his Sandringham estate, a set of jockeys' weighing scales were used to double check that every lord and lady who arrived at his house left a few pounds heavier on their departure.

Nowadays, Prince Charles is the most representative of the family trait, though he swings in a more fastidious direction. The royal catalog is rife with tales of his persnickety food standards. Like how, when once served a cup of tea at the White House (alas, with the tea bag still floating inside) he found himself paralyzed by bewilderment, unable to take a single sip. "I didn't know what to do with it," Charles admitted. Or how, when traveling abroad, his staff send out detailed instructions to hotel chefs in advance, outlining the precise "dimensions and texture" of his favorite sandwiches. Or how, when staying at Balmoral, he refuses to eat the local veggies, preferring to ship in all carrots and cabbages from his own garden at Highgrove, about 500 miles away. Royal biographers tend to blame Charles's nanny, Helen Lightbody, for instilling this astonishing fussiness. It's said she took pleasure in tormenting the Palace kitchen with her exacting standards. Dishes for young Charles were constantly being refused or remade based on little more than Nanny Lightbody's personal whims. The Queen eventually had enough and fired her.* And Elizabeth's own childhood offers clues to why.

For one, Elizabeth's mother held strong convictions about raising her daughters in an environment of simplicity. Coming from a rich,

---

* Apparently it came down to a pudding in the end. In 1956 the Queen sent the nursery a simple request that Charles, then eight years old, be given a special pudding she thought he might like. Nanny Lightbody refused, crossed the dessert from the menu, and incurred the Crown's wrath. Nobody crosses out the Queen's request.

though relaxed, Scottish family, the Queen Mother was raised on plain, wholesome country food. She never allowed the sumptuous luxury of wealth to go to the princesses' heads, or stomachs. There were occasions for treats (homemade fudge was a particular favorite), but Margaret and Elizabeth were mostly brought up on variations of "hoosh-mi," Margaret's made-up word for an endless variety of English nursery food, typically some nondescript mixture of meat, potatoes and gravy smooshed together—the sort of unpretentious fare the Queen has come to prefer. To this day, whenever Elizabeth is served a bowl of fresh strawberries for dessert, she automatically starts crushing them into a puree, in typical hoosh-mi fashion.

It's also difficult to ignore the influence the Second World War had on the Queen's attitude towards food. From an early teenager, Elizabeth saw a Britain racked by true scarcity. More food for the war effort meant tight rationing at home, restricting important staples to measly proportions. In 1940, 4 oz. of sugar, 2 oz. of butter and 2 oz. of cheese was one person's ration *per week.** It was a world in which the Tower of London's moat was converted into a vegetable patch to grow more food, where children chewed carrots in place of sweets and if you accidentally dropped an egg, you darn well scooped it up and scrambled it for dinner. Food was the fuel that was helping to win the war. To waste it, to think about food in frivolous ways, to overindulge when so many were going hungry seemed tantamount to a war crime. And in retrospect, such attitudes paid off. Many historians agree that the English during World War II were the healthiest they've ever been. It was a national experiment, a collective crash course in teaching the public how *not* to be drama-food-queens. Brits of the wartime generation are, by and large, totally incapable of fussing over food. The experiment worked. Though how well it has worked out for the Queen is worth exploring.

------

* The King insisted the royal family be put on the same ration plan. He also drastically cut all lights and heat used in royal residences and drew shallow lines around bathtubs to minimize hot water. And though Elizabeth claims she never went hungry or experienced great privation during the war, the austere experience left its mark.

*

If Elizabeth ever submitted to a round of testing by a dietary scientist (a wild thought, I grant you), she would likely emerge officially dubbed a "cool" thinker. Cool thinkers are people who put psychological distance between them and food. They typically see food as "just fuel" and are not prone to overthink or emote about their next meal. This is directly opposed to "hot" thinkers: people who look at food through a more visceral lens of feelings, past flavor memories and complicated emotions. Think Sarah Ferguson, Duchess of York, one of the more obsessive "hot" eaters in royal history. "With every smell, I smell food," she once admitted. "With every sight, I see food. I can almost hear food. I want to spade the whole lot through my mouth at Mach 2. Basta!"

The hot/cool distinction was first popularized by psychologist Walter Mischel, lead researcher of the now classic Stanford "marshmallow test." Studying self-control in preschoolers, Mischel noticed that children could successfully resist a food temptation (such as a large fluffy marshmallow) if they used cool, abstract thoughts to emotionally distance themselves from the tempting food. Visualizing the marshmallow as simply a soft, round object in a picture frame, for instance, worked wonders in increasing their resistance. In contrast, thinking "hot" thoughts, imagining how chewy and yummy and satisfying the marshmallow would be, almost guaranteed that the preschooler's willpower would snap. More recent studies, focusing on older age brackets, have confirmed the findings, as well as shone light on one of the baseline reasons why the vast majority of diets fail so quickly. If you're a hot thinker who hasn't learned to cool down your foodie thoughts, you'll eventually fall victim to the same cravings every time.*

From a purely anthropological point of view, it's interesting to note how many members of the English upper classes arrived at the same

---

* It mostly boils down to your brain's ability to override your good intentions. Research shows that merely thinking about a food in "hot" ways (how good it tastes, smells, looks) can trigger a chain of unintended Pavlovian reactions—namely, preempting your pancreas to secrete insulin, which lowers your blood sugar, which heightens feelings of hunger, which makes you more likely to give in to cravings whether you are truly hungry or not.

discovery independently. Traditionally surrounded by culinary abundance, adopting cooler thoughts towards food became a crucial survival mechanism among the higher echelons of British society. Top-drawer Brits weren't expected to care too deeply about the alimentary side of life. Displaying anything other than a nonchalant attitude towards their next nibble, in fact, was positively *déclassé*. As social historian Margaret Visser notes, *nonchalance* literally means achieving the state of "not being heated." Better British nannies than Helen Lightbody were on the front lines of inculcating this cooling detachment from an early age. Any sign of overt foodie-ness among aristo children was quickly nipped in the bud. Questions like "What's for lunch, Nanny?" were often given roundabout answers, such as "a rasher of wind and a fried snowball." The same went for "What's for pudding?"—"Patience pudding with a wait-a-while sauce," their nannies would reply. It eventually did the trick. In his compiled list of national eccentricities, the journalist Jeremy Paxman lists "indifference to food" as one of the hallmarks of essential Englishness, along with "village cricket . . . Shakespeare [and] country churches."

Newly relocated to England, American writer Sarah Lyall discovered just how alive the tendency still is. When invited to an *alfresco* lunch at the country estate of a rich earl, she imagined all sorts of conspicuous consumption in store: "wicker baskets, smoked salmon, asparagus, a babbling brook . . ." What emerged was a no-frills picnic of canned tomato soup served in Styrofoam cups and ham sandwiches on the commonest of white bread, all pulled from the back of a beat-up Jeep. The best of British *nonchalance* in action.

Likewise, if you're hankering for a gourmet cocktail reception, the best royalty can buy, you'll be far more comfortable at Clarence House (Prince Charles's London residence). There you'll be greeted by an exquisite assortment of beyond-organic hors d'oeuvres garnished with vegetables and posh herbs (very likely handpicked by the prince himself). If you simply want to meet the Queen, however, be prepared for some wine, a bowl of crisps and maybe, if you're lucky, some nuts at Buckingham Palace. Consider it an entry-level test. If you can confront the lackluster spread without complaining, you are one step closer to acting like a Queen. If your foodie-sensibilities are affronted, may I turn your attention to the first helpful piece of advice offered to American servicemen in Britain at the start of World War II: "NEVER criticize the King or Queen. Don't criticize the food."

QUEEN OF SCONES

OR RULE #2—TAKE TIME FOR TEA

One of the secrets of a happy life is continuous small treats.
—IRIS MURDOCH

I t's a glorious summer day in London. Gigantic tents are being hoisted over the pristine lawns of Buckingham Palace, and the general peasantry is pouring in. It's the most democratic event in the royal year, a massive meet and greet for 8,000 lucky subjects to be recognized by their monarch for various contributions to British society. Be you a global CEO, local baker or candlestick maker, if you get an invitation to Her Majesty's annual garden party, you don your best I-could-pass for a Middleton outfit and go running off for the royal lawn. For the chance to meet the Queen, of course, but everyone knows it's more about the buffet.

Whatever might be said for other lackluster food events at the Palace, when it comes to her garden party, the Queen goes all out. There's a designated tea tent straight out of *Alice in Wonderland*: 400 feet of the daintiest sandwiches, cakes and assorted pastries the eye has ever beheld, all of which the Queen has personally inspected for perfection. And if you haven't tasted Her Majesty's special blend of Darjeeling and Assam, you haven't lived, mate—or so go the bragging rights to last a lifetime.

But hang on . . . where *is* Her Majesty?

After thoroughly schmoozing the crowd, she appears to have completely bypassed the *Wonderland* tent—didn't even grab a quick finger sandwich—and is now sitting down with nary a watercress sprig to her name. The sight generally invokes comment on the Queen's fantastic feats of willpower, with perhaps a tinge of pity from ladies in starched hats who, after their fourth scone, are feeling quite regal and at home: *Poor dear, look at her sitting there, without a morsel between her lips, while persons of doubtful breeding clodhop over her beautiful lawn.*

But royal appearances can be deceiving. Contrary to popular myth, the Queen does *not* have superhuman willpower, she isn't interested in deprivation and really does enjoy all those exquisite delights from the tea tent. In fact, to find any record of the Queen "going without" is to rewind back to 1950, when Prince Philip helped Elizabeth lose a bit of pregnancy weight by encouraging her to give up potatoes and sweets for a while. At all other times in her long life, the Queen has eaten the food she enjoys, without any perceptible effect on her figure. The luck of good genes, you might think? Hardly. The walls of Windsor are packed with portraits of her tubby ancestors: most of them artfully concealing, at best, a triple chin. Queen Anne once ate what she jolly well liked too, resulting in such stupendous girth upon her death, she forever garnered the unhappy nickname of "Square Coffin" to future historians. Yet Elizabeth has escaped the family dilemma with seemingly little effort. Though if any real luck was involved in solving the problem, it was in the lucky way she stumbled upon the solution.

As a young girl, sitting at the dining room table with her family, Elizabeth realized something most adults still haven't grasped: treats were *more* enjoyable when she delayed eating them.

A little family ritual meant that after luncheon, the King would reach into his bowl of crystallized coffee sugar and offer his daughters a few pieces each. Margaret couldn't get the lumps of sugar into her mouth fast enough, but Elizabeth *liked* to delay. She first lined up the crystals on the table, in careful order of size, then ate them slowly, one by one. Elizabeth's governess Marion Crawford recounted the story in her memoirs to illustrate the seeds of self-restraint she saw in the little princess. Though if she lived today, Crawford would find her pupil little changed. The Queen is still theoretically lining up her sugar crystals. It just goes by another name now—the all-important ritual at the root of her famous restraint: teatime.

This is no mere "cup" of tea, a sloshing mug of caffeine to power-sip between meetings with cabinet ministers. Tea in the royal household is a borderline sacred tradition. For as long as she can remember, every afternoon at five, a kettle sings somewhere in the Queen's head, reminding her to temporarily close up shop. All work is put aside for a quiet hour, and she takes time to treat herself to her favorite meal. "In our family, everything stops for tea," says Prince Charles, one of his few food statements the Queen would heartily support. Because for all her culinary reserve, teatime is when the Queen lets loose.

*

Sitting beside a lace-lined cart of tiny sandwiches, cakes, gingerbread, muffins and scones, Elizabeth brews a silver pot of Darjeeling or Earl Grey, chatting with whatever royal relations are present. A snug quality of sameness pervades the scene. There's always the same Victorian teapot (refitted by Prince Philip to be self-boiling), the silver cow-shaped cream jug (an heirloom from William IV), the thin cucumber sandwiches shaped like octagons, the same ritualistic care Elizabeth takes in pouring out the tea, never allowing a single leaf to escape.* Closer to the realm of ceremony than afternoon snack, teatime for the Queen is "an exercise in grounding," writes biographer Carolly Erickson, "a calming and reassuring rite" of nonnegotiable importance. Every royal engagement in London is scheduled around it. Afternoon visits with the Queen religiously wrap up around four thirty, giving her just enough time to zip back to the Palace for tea. When Elizabeth travels farther abroad, a dedicated tea trunk accompanies her luggage, with supplies of China and Indian tea, along with fruitcake and shortbread biscuits, should teatime

---

* Despite the care involved, it's hardly a staid affair, and chuckles can frequently be heard over the clank of china. Especially when someone brings up the flying-cake incident. Years ago, a hapless footman had difficulty getting the wooden extension on the tea cart to open. He tampered with the gizmo a little too forcefully. The flap popped upon with force, catapulting a cream cake onto Her Majesty's chest—to roars of laughter.

emergencies arise. Her Majesty knows what she can handle, and a day without tea is not one of them.

Granted, this may look like an astonishing *lack* of willpower, if it wasn't so clever. Because far from evidence of the Queen's neediness, it shows how brilliantly she understands the workings of willpower itself. For as psychologists are discovering, willpower isn't the airy birthright of the virtuous, a skill to master or an inner power to harness. It's far more analogues to a muscle in your body: a mass of emotional energy that gets used, worn out, depleted and requires frequent rests to replenish itself. In laboratory experiments, people can be observed literally *using up* their willpower (mostly by resisting a tempting treat), which saps their self-control like a battery, leaving them unable to exert additional will-power for other non-food-related tasks.* "There's been more than two hundred studies on this idea," says Professor Mark Muraven, a leading researcher in the field of self-control. "Willpower isn't just a skill. It's a muscle, like the muscles in your arms or legs, and it gets tired as it works harder, so there's less power left over for other things." The accuracy of the analogy is most apparent when you consider the fact that your phys-ical muscles and mental willpower can be refueled by the same edible substance: glucose (a.k.a. sugar). In studies where people are expected to perform difficult brain exercises, those who are deprived of sugar during the process find their performance, determination and emotions all rapidly plummeting. "No glucose, no willpower," says psychologist Roy Baumeister.

The Queen's private secretaries, like Sir John Colville, like to remark that she carries out her endless round of duties "by sheer strength of willpower." But that is only partially true. Elizabeth does

---

* The first and most famous of these studies, conducted in 1996, involved sitting participants down before a table with two foods: a bowl of raw radishes and a bowl of deliciously aromatic cookies. Half the participants were allowed to help themselves to the cookies, half were told they could eat *only* the radishes. An agonizingly complicated puzzle was then set before them. Compared to the cookie eaters, who looked relaxed while working on the puzzle for long stretches of time, the radish eaters simply couldn't cope with the strain. They muttered and complained and quit the puzzle in bursts of temper. Exerting most of their willpower previ-ously resisting the cookies, little, if any, remained for higher matters.

have a seemingly inexhaustible spring of self-control to tap into, but only because she takes the time to replenish it. Her daily teatime habit is that crucial interval for recharging her willpower batteries, when her muscles of self-discipline relax and her personal weaknesses are indulged. For the Queen, this means getting the chance to temporarily glory in glucose: from the shortbread, the scones and the "jam pennies" (tiny raspberry jam sandwiches) she adores. However quaint it might sound, part of the secret to her unflappable personality is that she takes time for tea.

＊

All Britons thought along similar lines once, before dietitians ruined their intuition. An afternoon tea break—replete with their own cozy rituals—had positive effects on everyone's mood, and few were wont to give up the pleasure that got them sanely through the day. "Beneath simple roofs, the hour of tea has something in it of the sacred," wrote the novelist George Gissing in 1903, using words that could still describe the Queen's exact feelings today: "The mere chink of cups and saucers tunes the mind to happy repose." The idea that anyone would willingly forgo this treat was so inconceivably un-British, the future King Edward VII (infamous playboy though he was) once narrowly escaped getting entangled in a messy divorce case because of it. The Victorian public simply couldn't square the thought that anything as sordid as adultery could occur during the hallowed hour of teatime.

The legacy might account for why Elizabeth feels so much at home in Scandinavian countries, like Norway and Sweden, where the habit of enjoying an afternoon treat is still widely respected. Both countries encourage daily dips into what the Swedes call *fika*—a quiet pause in the day, a conscious decision to slow down over a warm beverage and a guilt-free smackerel of something sweet. In those cultures, to practice fika once a day simply marks you out as a stable, well-adjusted adult. "Life without fika is unthinkable," writes Swedish lifestyle expert Anna Brones. Fika even took on the status of "hot new food trend" in America a few years back, but for a country who has forgotten how and why to honestly treat themselves, it soon took on the form of an impossible gimmick. Surely Swedes couldn't indulge like this every day and still remain one of the slimmest populaces in Europe? It all seemed absurd. But the Queen has lived its reality for decades.

Researchers would likely attribute its success to a very counterintuitive mind-trick called "positive procrastination." You might expect that waiting to enjoy your slice of cake at teatime (or fika) would create such unbearable cravings of anticipation beforehand, once the tea cart finally arrived, you'd wind up eating the whole jar of clotted cream, just for starters. But the exact opposite occurs. Compared to people who strictly deny themselves certain pleasures, people who fully give themselves mental permission to indulge at a later opportunity (say, five o'clock at the Palace) naturally scale back their appetite when five o'clock eventually rolls around. Amazingly, it appears the brain derives the majority of its pleasure by simply giving itself *permission* to luxuriate at a later time, allowing you to arrive at that long-awaited treat with part of the craving already satisfied. It's essentially the same discovery Elizabeth made with the sugar crystals as a young girl: a pleasure postponed is sweeter. Subsequently, the actual amount of treats the Queen consumes at teatime has always remained small. As royal chronicler Brian Hoey explains, "even though every delicacy imaginable is available, the Queen eats sparingly and most of the goodies, especially the scones, get gobbled up by the corgis." The same goes for another teatime favorite at the Palace: Chocolate Biscuit Cake (little more than crushed tea biscuits molded inside layers of dark-chocolate ganache*). "The Queen is such a disciplinarian," says chef Darren McGrady, "it amazed me that we would send a great big chocolate cake up . . . at afternoon tea, and she would just take the tiniest slice." The cake is nibbled down gradually, a little every day, "until there is only one tiny piece [left]," adds McGrady. "But you have to send that up. She wants to finish the whole of that cake!"

Any diet based on denying yourself that "tiny piece" has never worked. It never worked for royalty either. Queen Victoria spent her childhood in a near-constant state of gustatory denial. She was allowed only the dullest, scantiest meals and, as a result, took every opportunity to gorge when no one was looking—a dysfunctional eating pattern,

---

* Chocolate Biscuit Cake is such a perennial hit among the royal family, it was chosen as the groom's cake for William and Catherine's wedding breakfast in 2011.

accompanied by escalating weight gain, that followed her the rest of her life. More recently, Sarah Ferguson freely admits to doing "the craziest things to lose weight" during her royal career, vacillating between all-out restrictions (like the meat-and-oranges diet she lived on before her wedding to Prince Andrew) to all-out binges of her favorite indulgences (like cheese, mayonnaise and tomato sandwiches)—dieting swings which earned her the unfair, but perhaps inevitable, title of "Duchess of Pork" in the press. As Brian Wansink explains in *Mindless Eating*, "If we consciously deny ourselves something again and again, we're likely to end up craving it more and more. . . . The foods we don't bite can come back to bite us."

There's an insightful story of Elizabeth trying to persuade Margaret to heed a similar piece of advice: not to deny, simply to delay. At a garden party when both were young, Margaret, chomping at the bit to get to the refreshments, had to be gently instructed by her older sister in the proper ways of princesses: "You must *not* be in too much of a hurry to get through to the crowds to the tea table. That's not polite." Polite or just plain practical, the Queen can fully relax at her garden parties today because of it. While onlookers gawk at her willpower, she knows the crowds will soon disperse and five o'clock will find her sitting snug beside her own familiar tea pot, recharging her willpower batteries. And if there's any tinge of pity going around, it's for the guests who gave up a once-in-a-lifetime chance to meet their monarch in order to get a bounding head start on the buffet—otherwise known as the poor dears who never learned how to properly take time for tea.

Tiaras if Possible

or Rule #3—Manners maketh
moderation

*Table manners, which constitute proof positive that the people
employing them are not "like beasts," have always set out
to make eating not easier but . . . more difficult.*
—Margaret Visser, *The Rituals of Dinner*

"I could eat all that!" said the woman with the movie star body,
pointing at an entire cherry cheesecake and several pizzas
behind the cafeteria's glass display. She drew the food in with
her magnetic blue eyes, just as she drew in the photographers around
her. "It doesn't matter what I eat," she told the admiring press, "I never
put an ounce on!" Her stunning figure, so richly endowed with fairy-tale
glamour, made it almost seem possible. Perhaps, just this once, the fairy
tale was true.

The woman was Princess Diana and, sadly, nothing was further
from it. The same press corps soon discovered the harsher reality:
Diana's tragic reliance on the quick fix of bulimia that imprisoned her
in a vicious cycle of cravings, binges and compulsive trips to the loo.
She never put a perceptible "ounce on" because she never saw another
realistic way to have her cake and keep her iconic figure. But the peripheral tragedy was that there *was* another way. An entire philosophical
approach to food was already in place at the Palace for achieving a very
similar goal, albeit with far more bodily grace.

21

It once went by the illustrious umbrella term of "courtesy," originally practiced, as it was, by medieval noblemen at *court*. The nobility were the ones who needed it most: people of unshackled privilege who required precise boundaries to live by. Ironically, Diana's ancestors were among the class who formulated its rules—rules which, when attended to, would help anyone cope with the excesses of life though mindfulness and moderation. They're still carefully observed at Elizabeth's court today, though you probably know them better as *table manners*.

If you were expecting something more profound, I grant you, the term has seen better days. Table manners have been all but banished to the frilly realms of comic relief—cue Anne Hathaway strapped to a dining room chair in *The Princess Diaries*, a Hermès scarf straitjacketing her from reaching, too impolitely, for the saltshaker. The visuals don't get much better for real-life royals either. It wasn't too long ago when Queen Mary (Elizabeth's grandmother) refused to touch any foods with her fingers and made a point of arriving at every dinner in the full regalia of evening dress and tiara, even when dining alone. Another stickler, Princess Alice of Athlone—Victoria's oldest-surviving granddaughter—saw sweeping changes to Palace etiquette during her day, but she was still issuing birthday invitations into the 1970s with the friendly reminder to her guests: "tiaras if possible." This rather excludes, well, everyone who didn't inherit said diamond-encrusted doodad, which hasn't exactly made Palace etiquette feel relevant for those of the TNP (tiaras not possible) persuasion. But take it from Elizabeth, a woman who spends less time in her tiara and more time surrounded by the sort of bountiful spreads most of us experience only at office holiday parties, table manners can be your saving grace.

Because in spite of snobs everywhere—people who glory in earth-shattering etiquette debates, like whether the pudding spoon goes above or beside the dinner plate—when whittled down to their original roots, good manners remain our easiest tool for approaching meals more moderately. First created by people who needed physical limits in life, table manners function like prandial speed bumps, reminding us to resist the natural urge to plow through our meals, as the Duchess of York would say, at "Mach 2." More primitively, they reinforce the always necessary nudge that we aren't savage animals and shouldn't eat like them. Anthropologist Kate Fox demystified the matter best in her seminal fieldwork observing English eaters in action. Condensing hundreds of individual rules on etiquette, she noticed that much of what the English consider "good manners" at the table—especially among the upper classes—revolve around the adherence of two simple concepts, what she calls the "small is beautiful" and "slow is beautiful" principles. Both are widely practiced at the Palace and make up the majority of the Queen's direct daily interaction with food.

※

Take the concept of slowness. Behind practically every do and don't in the panoply of table manners is a sneaky design to limit the rate at which food enters one's mouth. Bread is a prime example. According to Palace protocol, the usual method of cutting a roll in two, slathering both sides with butter and chomping merrily away is too efficient, too quick, too mindless—and therefore too boorishly wrong. "I didn't know you didn't eat the bread roll like that," admitted Claire Foy during an interview for *The Crown*, mouthing a massive pretend bite to show what not to do. Her queenly training simply wasn't complete without learning the proper *breadiquette*.

One works gracefully through the roll instead, breaking off one bite-sized morsel at a time and buttering *only* that individual piece—pop in mouth and repeat the sequence, if desired. The fact that you might well be compelled to stop (probably by the early onset of carpal tunnel) halfway through the roll is entirely the point. Manners maketh moderation.*

Even the Queen's cutlery helps to achieve this—or more correctly, how she holds it. Rather than grasping the fork in her right hand, tines facing up, taking full advantage of the forks curved ability to scoop up a hearty mouthful (otherwise known as "how the crass Americans do it"),

---

* This care also extends to tea, and how to properly stir it. Crucial, this, if you're ever invited to the Palace and want to leave with your dignity intact. A cup of tea should never be stirred in a circular motion (because sugar dissolves too vulgarly fast that way) but with gentle back and forth sweeps of the spoon. If the cup were a clock, think silently striking the twelve and six position repeatedly.

the Queen prefers a purposefully slower technique. As a proponent of the politer, European-style of eating, the fork is transferred into her left hand, the knife into her right, opening up whole new worlds of ineffi- ciency. Since forks, when held upright, are too spiky for polite society (the medieval memory of impaling devices is still a bit strong among the aristocracy), every bite that can't be easily speared must be carefully coaxed and cajoled onto the *back* of the fork and brought to the mouth, tines demurely facing down, without spillage. English etiquette books are full of helpful—if somewhat sanity-questioning—tips on managing this without social embarrassment, especially when it comes to peas. (N.B. If your fellow diners start visibly perspiring when confronted with a dish of garden-variety peas, you know you're in an upper-class English household.) But moderation, again, is at the root. "Denying a modern fork its possible spoonlike use" might be "wantonly perverse," says etiquette historian Margaret Visser, but the technique "forces us to take small mouthfuls and to leave some of the food, unliftable, on the plate. It is difficult to get the food onto the fork, and harder still to balance and raise it faultlessly. Managing to eat like this with grace is a triumph of practice and determination."

Thankfully, Elizabeth goes easy on the unpracticed.* Guests at royal dinners usually find foods cut conveniently small. *Delicate* is the watch- word for every dish set before the Queen. Alluding to this unspoken rule as he carefully paired down a handful of green beans to a more refined size, former royal chef Graham Newbould once remarked, "You can't be seen with beans hanging out of your mouth. . . . It's got to be quite delicate." But in her appreciation for the petite, Elizabeth is showing her true understanding of luxury. The Greek word for "luxu- rious living"—*tryphe*—doesn't connote copious quantities of food or the eater's prerogative to binge until he barfs. Instead, as Margaret Visser notes, *tryphe* comes from a verb meaning "to crumble or reduce

---

* Like the time during one luncheon at the Palace when a nervous guest proved no match for an uncooperative potato. It slipped off his plate and rolled onto the floor, where he strained every muscle in his foot to demurely prevent the spud from rolling farther before, alas, it was squashed all the same. "Life can be so difficult," whispered the Queen, secretly watching the whole time.

to fragments." Only the rich could crumble away their time, reducing foods to dainty morsels, thereby showing the less socially fortunate they didn't have to rush or stuff to survive—habits which formed the bedrock of Western table manners. The Queen can still be observed keeping up the custom . . . anytime she eats a banana. She must *reduce* it first, using a fork and knife to cut off both ends, make a slit down the middle and slice the inner fruit into small rounds, which she also eats with a fork (this is obviously opposed to the peel-and-scarf technique observable in monkeys). As anthropologist Kate Fox would argue, "small is beautiful" to the well born.*

Failure to understand this principle was one of the many, *many* reasons Wallis Simpson collided with royal protocol in the 1930s. (She's "that woman" Edward VIII abdicated the throne for.) Let's just say her big plans to Americanize the menu at Balmoral with supersized triple-decker sandwiches wasn't met with rounds of unadulterated applause. It also accounts for the awkward time once had by the Queen Mother in the 1950s, during a round of formal diplomatic dinners in America. A woman of impeccable English manners, she was dumbfounded by the portion sizes across the pond. Writing to her daughter Elizabeth on the occasion, "I have never hated anything so much as the two big dinners. . . . It really is a nightmare, & they give one gigantic bits of meat, bigger than this sheet of paper."

Elizabeth would have readily sympathized. Good manners, coupled with a strong aversion to waste has instilled her with a lifelong preference for small portions too. This means that—in a fabulous reversal of historic royal dining habits—when the Queen dines with guests, she'll typically wind up with the smallest serving on offer. "If she were being served steak," said a former Palace official, "we would make sure the Queen got the smallest piece." Henry VIII would have beheaded anyone cheeky enough to propose the idea, but Elizabeth II likes it that way. She

---

* Luxury tends to bring out the daintier eater in everyone—a trait happiness researcher Gretchen Rubin identifies as "consumption snobbery." Whether it's an expensive bottle of wine or a costly block of imported cheese, people consume things with purposefully smaller bites and sips if they pay more for the items or, likewise, find themselves in more elegant surroundings.

also prefers to serve herself from salvers passed around the table, rather than be given a plate with an allocated portion size already determined by someone else in the kitchen. It gives her more control. She'll help herself to a small portion to start, then return for seconds, if necessary. "That's the etiquette," says chef Graham Newbould. "It's better to eat everything that you've got on your plate and ask for a little more, if you want some, rather than leave some."* Manners have taught the Queen, like her mother before her, to take meals at a nibble, not a gulp.

✳

The result is a Queen who has learned to recognize when she's full, and when to put her knife and fork down—a skill which isn't as commonplace as it sounds, especially in adults. And yet, we are all born with the same ability. No matter how much food you set before a group of three-year-olds, they'll naturally self-regulate their intake, stopping the moment their bodies tell them they've had enough, no matter how much food is left. In a few years, however, the instinct shows signs of weakening. Researchers have noticed that five-year-olds are more likely to eat according to external clues, like the size of an allocated portion, stopping when the portion is gone (not when they've reached a personal level of satiety). Picked up early, the habit follows the majority of Americans into adulthood. Many of us forget to stop the conveyor belt of feeding if more food remains on our plates.** Which is why table manners have

---

* The Queen is staunchly opposed to what political commentator Andrew Marr calls "the throwaway society." There are sheets and blankets and copper cooking pots still used at the Palace dating from the reign of Queen Victoria. Elizabeth gets years' worth of mileage out of her suitcases and riding gear, her shoes are reheeled when they wear down and she once sent Prince Charles back out into the grounds to look for a dropped dog lead (leash), reasoning, "Dog leads cost money."

** The French, by contrast, have largely escaped this fate, a cultural distinction first noticed by the pioneer of mindless eating research, Brian Wansink. Questioning both French and American diners about how they knew when to stop eating, the French reported that feelings of fullness were their main indicator while the Americans largely reported stopping a meal when their plate was empty or when the television show they were watching was over.

been so singularly successful in turning the Queen into a more mindful eater. With their speed limits of sophisticated rules, they slow down her meals, creating necessary pauses in between bites, allowing her body (not just her eyes) time to dictate when she's had enough. On one hand, this etiquette of *conscious deceleration* hides a wise biological fact. It takes twenty minutes for the stomach to tell the brain it's had enough. But the wisdom comes sharpest into focus when you consider its similarities to a custom practiced by one of the longest-lived populations in the world.

The Japanese are traditionally advised to begin (and sometimes end) every meal with the almost prayerlike utterance of *hara hachi bu*. Roughly translated as "belly 80-percent full," it's a reminder to eat and enjoy whatever nourishment is before them but to stop feasting just before they reach capacity—essentially to put down their chop-sticks when their bellies feel about 80 percent full. Culturally, eating by this ancient Confucian maxim is just good etiquette (similar to the avoidance of greed in Western table manners), but it's also been a mass demonstration of what happens when people consciously include their stomachs in mealtime decision-making. Longevity experts now consider the practice of *hara hachi bu* to be one of the key components behind the Japanese's iconically long life-spans.*

Whether she's familiar with the term or not, the Queen best demonstrated the heart of *hara hachi bu* when, rather fittingly, she was floating around another Pacific island. On her first Commonwealth tour in 1953, during a stop on the island of Tonga, Elizabeth was greeted by the hefty Queen Salote, who threw a colossal feast for her and 700 hungry guests, all of whom were sitting cross-legged on palm mats and eating with their fingers. With consummate tact, Elizabeth knelt down and dug in with the best of them, but was eventually seen easing up. While those around her were still busy picking away at the endless portions of roast pig, her etiquette training kicked in. As the highest person of rank, she couldn't technically stop eating (or *everyone* would have to

---

* Explanations often focus on the biological consequences of IGF-1 (insulin-like growth factor 1)—a hormone with strong links to the aging process. Habitually eating beyond the point of fullness is thought to increase levels of IGF-1, thereby heightening the presence of damaging oxidative stress in the body.

stop), but she knew when enough was enough. "So out of consideration for others," remembers then lady-in-waiting Pamela Mountbatten, "she had to play with her food and [pretend to] extend the time eating," without actually taking another bite.

Consideration for others is traditionally offered as the prime objective for adopting better manners today. But consideration for your own limits is an equally important reason. The ancient term "courtesy" extends both ways, to others and to self. It certainly has for the Queen. She's never been interested in casual dining, if "casual" is taken literally—something that happens by accident or chance, meals that could leave her a "causality" of mindless consumption.* Because even when she's not dinning in exotic locales or off of gold plates at State Banquets, when her schedule is clear and when she's all alone—just her and a little supper tray in her private apartment—manners are still present, helping to moderate every bite.

---

* A conviction she lives up to linguistically as well. Elizabeth refuses to use the casual term "lunch" when referring to her midday meal. She thinks it sounds too "vulgar," says royal chronicler Brian Hoey. More correctly, only *luncheon* is served at the Palace. "I am the last bastion of standards," admits the Queen.

THE WINDSOR
WETS' CLUB

OR RULE #4—DRINK LIKE
YOU REIGN IT

The answer, if you ask me, is that the Queen Mum
has a reputation for liking her drop of gin. Everyone loves a granny,
but a granny on the razzle is irresistible.

—PLAYWRIGHT KEITH WATERHOUSE, EXPLAINING THE QUEEN MOTHER'S POPULARITY

B uckingham Palace has never had a problem attracting new
workers. The pay might be considerably lower than the national
average, but there's a peripheral bundle of perks to cash in on
for those employed in Her Majesty's household. Highest on the list is
what a stint at the Palace does for a resume: virtually any door of future
employment swings wide open. Coming a close second is the chance
to take a dip in the same swimming pool Prince Philip uses. But on
a day-to-day basis, nothing beats access to free meals from the royal
kitchen or the employees' drinking plan. In a perk that often surprises
outsiders, there's a subsidized staff bar at the Palace with dirt-cheap gin
and tonics and other bevys daily up for grabs. By decree of the boss
lady at the top, kicking back with a well-deserved tipple is practically a
human right.

With a knowing clink to the glass, anyone familiar with the House
of Windsor's attitude toward alcohol would expect nothing less. The

family has never concealed the fact that they appreciate a stiff one now and again. In the jazzy heydays of the 1930s, the Queen Mother went so far as to form a less-than-secret drinking society among friends, with her as acting patroness. Known as the Windsor Wets' Club, they had cryptic signs, proposed matching neckties and a half-joking motto that went *aqua vitae non aqua pura*. If I may take liberties in translating: water is wimpy, liquor is quicker. Years later, and well into her nineties, there was still a visible twinkle in the Queen Mother's eye whenever anyone proposed a nip of her favorite bracer. "I hear you like gin?" said one nervous hostess, unsure what to offer a visiting royal. "I hadn't realized I enjoyed that reputation," replied the Queen Mother, sweetly feigning shock. "But as I do, perhaps you could make it a large one."

Lines like that have given rise to some pretty tall tales about the level of libating going on at the Palace. If you believe internet gossip, Elizabeth outmatches her mother's self-avowed "drinking powers" by habitually knocking back four strong cocktails a day—starting just before luncheon. Apparently mincing about in an alcoholic miasma throughout the day, the Queen is said to turn a relaxed eye away from members of her household who occasionally overdo it on the sherry and shenanigans themselves. Like the time Elizabeth supposedly found a drunk servant sprawled at the bottom of a staircase. Without putting a pearl out of place, she merely requested to anyone within earshot, "Would someone please come and pick Frank up, I think he's a little under the weather."*

Such stories send the press into giddy hysterics, competing over who can pen the most cutesy headline—"All the Queen's Gin Couldn't Put the Palace Page Together Again"—but they are usually full of blatant misunderstandings and outright exaggerations. "She'd be pickled if she drank" as much as the media says she does, said royal chef Darren McGrady, setting the record straight on his former employer. But in our age of hyper-suspiciousness for anything remotely resembling a pleasurable substance, how the Queen values and, more importantly,

---

* Prince Philip only fanned the alcoholic flames when, in 1999, he was presented with a gift basket of Southern foods by the US ambassador. He spent a few seconds digging through the contents before undiplomatically inquiring, "Where's the Southern Comfort?"

uses alcohol for certain ends requires a bit of unraveling to appreciate its wisdom. To start, you could say she's spent a lifetime judiciously drinking under Sir Winston Churchill's famous maxim: *She has taken more out of alcohol than alcohol has taken out of her.*

❋

Elizabeth's real relationship with the bottle, if she has one, could be described as almost medicinal in nature. Throughout her reign, alcohol has always served in the function of fast-acting stress reliever—a dose of liquid decompression on hectic days. Hence her readiness to take a nip from the flask of brandy proffered by the Archbishop on her wedding day, to steady her nerves. Or her appreciation of a well-earned drink at the end of an emotional day suppressing tears during a World War II memorial. "The Queen's eyes were brimming," recalled a lady-in-waiting, who watched Elizabeth retreat into the Palace after the event, where "she quickly took a large gin and tonic and knocked it back." Elizabeth also rarely missed her Sunday afternoon date with the Queen Mother at Royal Lodge. After church, sipping a gin and Dubonnet with "Mummy" was one of her favorite ways to de-stress after a long week.

If this sounds like the slippery spiral of alcoholism, you might want to reconsider. Evidence of drinking patterns in "blue zones" around the world (places where life expectancies are much higher than average) reveal a very similar approach to alcohol. Places like Sardinia, Italy, Ikaria, Greece, and Okinawa, Japan—where it isn't uncommon to see 100-year-olds walking down the street—all place cultural value on softly winding down the day with a hard drink. As longevity expert Dan Buettner explains, drawing on his firsthand research into "blue zone" lifestyles, one of the most overlooked benefits to this traditional way of drinking isn't always found in the usual explanation of red wine's healthy antioxidants (the Japanese are sake drinkers, after all) but in something more universal: "it may also be that a little alcohol at the end of the day reduces stress," says Buettner, "which is good for overall health."

Aside from a well-working liver, this could be the best explanation for why alcohol was more helpful than harmful in the Queen Mother's life, extended to the ripe old age of 101. Drinks punctuated her day into ritualized periods of relaxation. "She loved social drinking," says

Major Colin Burgess, serving as the Queen Mother's equerry for two years, who recorded a typical day in the life of this regally "devoted drinker." She'd start at noon with a gin and Dubonnet with a slice of lemon and lots of ice, followed by a glass of red wine at luncheon. Then came what she called "the magic hour" at six o'clock, when she deemed herself deserving of a dry martini, chased by a glass of champagne (or two) at dinner. The almost affectionate tag of the Queen Mother having "hollow legs" was perhaps inevitable. And a pub-going British public loved her for it, especially when they discovered that she liked to attend horse races with a thermos secretly filled with champagne. "It's one of my little treats," she explained with a mischievous grin. But her drinking "habit" was just that: a pattern, a predictable routine she clearly derived pleasure and relaxation from. That it became a drinking *problem* "was simply unimaginable," said her closest niece, Margaret Rhodes, clearing up rumors in her memoirs. "Her alcohol intake never varied." There were no days of binging, she said. "There was no excess." The Queen Mother was a "steady" drinker, says royal historian Adrian Tinniswood, rather than an "excessive" one.*

Going above your established personal limit is the only thing that will ever worry a Windsor.

There's a fabulous story of the Queen Mother lunching with her daughter when Elizabeth asked for another glass of wine, exceeding her usual single standard. "Now, now, Lilibet," implored her mother with a mock frown. "Remember, you have to reign all afternoon." She was preaching to the smartest woman in the proverbial pub. Time and again, Elizabeth has demonstrated the virtue of drinking with her unique purpose in mind, moderating her alcohol consumption based on who she is and what she is on earth for. As the visible head of state, knowing that practically any hour might summon her need for a clear

---

* Indeed one bottle the Queen Mother turned to most wasn't alcoholic at all: Malvern water. An entire book could be written about the royal family's obsession for this spring water from the Malvern Hills. Princess Margaret once argued (rather implausibly) that no other water on earth deserved the name. "Water is NOT water," she once said, schooling a confused host who tried offering her tap. "This . . . is water," said Margaret, pointing to a bottle of Malvern she brought with her. "Now do you see what I mean?"

head and sharp conversational skills, royal biographers have found her to be almost "abstemious" on typical days at the Palace. Thanks to epic family fails in recent history, Elizabeth knows that sozzled monarchs don't last long in the job.* Hence one glass of pink vermouth and soda can last her through an entire cocktail party. At banquets, her glasses of assorted wine (one for each course) are likewise hardly touched, and if you see the Queen holding what looks like a substantial gin and tonic at a royal event, it could often be little more than plain tonic in the glass. In other words, she drinks like a woman who still has to reign over her personal kingdom.

Elizabeth shows every sign of being what, in behavioral psychology, is called a "self-transcendent" drinker: someone who adjusts her alcoholic intake according to values and duties bigger than herself. And though it may sound airy-fairy on the surface, self-transcendent drinking (or eating) appears to be a natural reflex anyone can tap into to help moderate their own libating habits. Specifically, researchers have noticed that people who think about their bigger life values, like their role in the community or helping others, before they take a bite or sip of something pleasurable, automatically self-regulate and often reduce their consumption of those things that would normally be hard to resist. On a grander scale, the tendency to look at alcohol through a bigger lens of personal, familial and cultural priorities may be why countries with a strong "drinking culture" have so few reported alcoholics. The French consistently rank as one of the highest consumers of alcohol in Europe, but France lists only slightly over one AA group per million persons in the entire country. Compare that to the hundreds of AA groups in New York City alone.

Drinking with more purpose brings crystal clarity to a substance designed to leave us anything but mentally clear, helping us determine when to abstain, when to judiciously sip and when to pour ourselves a jolly big one. In 1993 when Elizabeth heard that the prime minister

---

* Her uncle David's legitimate drinking problem was another chink in the poor choices that eventually cost him the throne in 1936. Observers recounted how footmen would stand behind him at meals, constantly refilling his glasses of wine until he was, in Palace vernacular, hardly fit to govern a tennis court.

of Australia, Paul Keating, strongly wished to turn the country into a republic, deeming a far-off monarch no longer necessary, the Queen knew exactly which moment was before her. Stating with all priorities fully considered, "Now I really do need a very large drink."

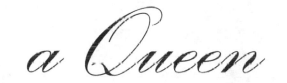

Work Like a Queen

My castle, my rules.

—*The King's Speech*

I t should have been the world's worst Christmas present. In 1928 Lady Airlie gave the then three-year-old Princess Elizabeth the bizarrely prosaic gift of a dustpan and brush for the holidays, no doubt under a cloud of disingenuous *how thoughtfuls!* from the attended royals. Yet whatever the gift said for Lady Airlie's frightful lack of creativity, it turned out to be more preparatory and prophetic that anyone could imagine. The dustpan and brush were emblems of work: daily, plodding, never-ending work. And after a series of family tragedies—an uncle who abdicated and a father who died too young—Elizabeth the Queen would soon come to know exactly what that entailed.

It's one of the biggest paradoxes of British royalty: as the Crown has steadily lost real power over the centuries, its wearer's workload and public responsibilities have increased exponentially. Essentially, less beheadings, more parliamentary paper work—a legacy Elizabeth has inherited at its most historically demanding zenith. The amount of work she voluntarily assumes is staggering. On her ninetieth birthday—and already 25 years past Britain's once mandatory retirement age—editors at the *Telegraph* didn't hesitate in naming her "the hardest worker of us all." There was a time when the energy of youth might have explained it, like how the Queen hit the ground running after her coronation, fulfilling a remarkable 500 royal engagements in her first year on the throne. But it can't account for how that number has barely budged over the decades. At age 82 Elizabeth was still logging 417 engagements in one year, occasions that keep her practically sprinting from one visit (school, community center, foreign country) to the next while hosting some 50,000 people in various receptions and ceremonies throughout the year. And *that* is only the Queen's public duties. In private, every day of the year, large red boxes are set on the Queen's desk bursting with parliamentary reports, foreign cables, intelligence documents and weekend dispatches from the Commonwealth to be carefully read through—a daily endeavor which takes roughly three hours to complete and breaks for only two days out of the entire year. Unlike almost every other worker in the world who can call it quits after a hard day at the office, the Queen is never off duty. On the throne, in the bath or in bed, she has been the boss of Britain everywhere, every hour, for over 65 years of her life, and counting.

"Playing at king is no sinecure," George IV observed with exhaustion, shocked by the daily grind of monarchy, a workload that has either made or broken his successors. The Queen Mother was convinced that the appropriately named *burden of kingship* killed her husband, Bertie, denying him the quiet country life he was destined for before Edward VIII abdicated. Anxiety-ridden and plagued by a debilitating stammer, Bertie was ill-equipped to handle the increasing public rigors of modern monarchy, coping through ceaseless rounds of cigarettes and late nights of work that contributed to his early death at age 56.* "He literally died for England," said his private secretary. Alan Bennett put it just about perfect in his play *The Madness of George III*, when he noted, "To be heir to the throne is not a position; it is a predicament." Princess Margaret expressed the same sentiment, albeit in humbler nursery jargon, when she first realized that her uncle's abdication meant her sister would one day become Queen. Turning to Elizabeth, Margaret could only utter a commiserating, "Poor you." Practically every person in the line of accession (however far removed) has gone on record stating as much. Prince Harry recently asked, "Is there any one of the royal family who wants to be king or queen? I don't think so." Currently a distant sixth in line to the throne, Harry is still taking no chances and has since scuttled off to North America in semiretirement.

Queen Mary worried long and hard about what the royal burden would do, one day, to her beloved granddaughter Elizabeth. The Windsors, up until then, hadn't seemed to be coping very well. One of her sons outright refused the job (Edward VIII), another gradually broke under its enormous strain (George VI). Little wonder she wrote, "I only

---

* Understandably, Elizabeth was adamant that Philip give up the habit that wreaked her father's health. Previously a heavy smoker himself, Philip obliged with phenomenal efficiency, going from a pack a day to quitting cold turkey on his wedding day.

hope they will not kill the poor little girl [Elizabeth] with overwork." Fortunately, never were genuine fears so unfounded. Not only has Elizabeth risen to the increasing modern challenges of the Crown, she has accepted more work, plowed through more red boxes, shaken more hands and visited more countries than any of her predecessors, without once buckling under the pressure. The promise she made in her first Christmas broadcast, in 1953, wasn't just a pleasantry tossed to the radio winds, but a lifelong vow to "give myself heart and soul" to her duties "every day of my life." At an age when most people are usually winding down their remaining days over a bingo table, Elizabeth is still keeping that vow, recently working over 40 hours a week and giving off what essayist Tom Nairn called, "an apparently inexhaustible electric charge." But as we'll explore in the following pages, it's a charge energized by *taking charge*, organizing her working life in ways that work best for her. Collectively known as "the Liz Biz," it can leave others equally inspired and dizzy in its wake.* As one journalist accurately observed, to spend any time with the Queen is to inevitably meet her "firm level gaze," which almost seems to say, "I've done my boxes—have you done yours?"

---

* Consider Catherine Middleton, whose employment status was noticeably vague before her engagement to Prince William. Yet almost immediately after meeting the Queen, her working life jump-started as an assistant buyer for the clothing store Jigsaw. It aligned with what Lady Joseph, wife of British stateman Keith Joseph, once told biographer Christopher Andersen: "The Queen doesn't expect the people around her to work as hard as she does. But she does expect them to work."

MOST EXCELLENT
ORDER OF ORDER
OR RULE #5—LISTEN TO
YOUR INNER BOBO

*This sense of order was, I found, very strong
in the family of my new employers.*
—MARION CRAWFORD, GOVERNESS TO ELIZABETH II

At the risk of sounding like a character out of *Mary Poppins*,
if you want to understand the Queen's unique working style,
you'll need to start by enlisting the services of a proper British
nanny—at least theoretically. Royal nannies like Clara Knight and
Margaret MacDonald (affectionately dubbed "Allah" and "Bobo" in the
nursery) were the sun and moon to Elizabeth's early days, ruling figures
of predictable routines as certain and reassuring as the seasons. Both
women held unmovable opinions on the importance of order and the
regularity of daily, repetitive schedules, especially Bobo, an old-school
Scotswoman. Hence every day like clockwork, Elizabeth would be
wheeled out in her pram or summoned to supper or put on the potty
in the unchanging orbit of nursery life. Heaven help a bowel movement that defied Bobo's timetable. Or Queen Mary's, for that matter.
It was her command the nannies were following, after all. Queen Mary
believed so strongly in the well-ordered life, she often went above her
more relaxed daughter-in-law's jurisdiction, reminding the nannies in

41

charge that "apart from even the question of health, one does feel that a punctual regular life is so essential for children." It was a life bound by limits. But Elizabeth thrived within its boundaries.

She loved living within this structured chrysalis with just enough room for *a time and place for everything*. Accounts from her childhood reveal how voluntarily she chose order over chaos. On Christmas and birthdays, rather than strew the gift wrapping and ribbons around the room, she carefully folded the paper and furbelows, storing them for another use. Her governess, "Crawfie," also observed the neat way Elizabeth lined up her toy horses at the end of the day, as well as her nightly displays of precision when it came to arranging her clothes and shoes on a nearby chair, sometimes jumping out of bed just to make sure her shoes were placed perfectly parallel to one another. To her father, these habits were little more than childish "fretwork" (what we might call OCD today) and Princess Margaret could always get the nursery staff giggling by imitating her sister's bedtime proclivities for popping out of the covers to rearrange her shoes. But in retrospect, they were the building blocks upon which much of the Queen's future success would depend.

As the CEO of what is sometimes called the royal "Firm," Elizabeth's early appreciation of order allowed her to take on a role inherently weighted by strict regimens and daily protocols. It's a bit like, as Princess Diana later described, always having to turn up on time for a wedding "every day of your life—as the bride." Yet what others might consider restrictive, the Queen found "strength in," says biographer Carolly Erickson, "adapting her [old nursery] habits to the rigid timetables, time-honored routines and somewhat archaic procedures of the longstanding palace establishment." From practically her first day as Queen, she slipped into a routine that has hardly varied over the years. There's always been a wake-up cup of Earl Grey at seven thirty, a prebreakfast bath, pouring over multiple newspapers at breakfast, mornings spent in meetings or sifting through her red boxes, afternoon visits outside the Palace, back in time for tea and the reading of more parliamentary reports, a possible cocktail reception or public dinner, then in bed by eleven o'clock with her journal and, possibly, a favorite book.

The royal year also revolves around a similar progress of predict-ability. "Almost every year, season by season, almost exactly the same things must be done, said and performed," says political commen-tator Andrew Marr—from public moments, like the Queen's speech at the Opening of Parliament and her annual televised broadcast at Christmas, to private movements, like her holiday pilgrimages to Balmoral and Sandringham. Indeed anyone who wishes to follow the Queen throughout the year need only consult the "Court Circular," a daily-published Palace bulletin imbued with an ingenious double meaning: wait long enough and royal life tends to repeat itself in *circular* patterns.

*

In our current novelty-addicted culture, it may be difficult to under-stand how this sort of constancy can be a virtue, but it has always been so for the British monarchy. In Tudor times, Elizabeth I proudly summarized her entire rule under the heraldic motto *Semper Eadem*: "always the same." Change for the sake of change has never been advan tageous for what is now the longest-continuous institution in English history.* A woman whose very soul embodied the maxim, the Queen Mother was always quick to spot the pointless idiocy of modern flash masquerading as progress. At the dawn of the new millennium, when Prime Minister Tony Blair sought to snazz up the country's image with his "Cool Britannia" marketing campaign, the Queen Mother could only look on in pity as the epically *uncool* campaign rolled out to a less than impressed public. "Poor Britannia," the Queen Mother remarked to a friend. "She would have hated being Cool." Because as Tony Blair failed to realize (he clearly wasn't raised by a nanny), constancy and predicable sameness can be incredibly grounding. It was a "lesson" the Duchess of York, Sarah Ferguson, had to learn "the hard way." After her wildly erratic career as the royal who was going to liven up the Palace

---

* King James I (1566–1625) liked to demonstrate the changeless stability of monarchy on a mythical scale. During courtly masques at the Palace of Whitehall, allegories in the form of Chaos and Corruption would run amok in the performance until, in the second half, the world was brought to order by the King himself.

with Fergie-filled fun and froth, Sarah found herself bouncing from one unforeseen scandal to the next until destructive publicity and sheer exhaustion made her desire firmer footing. These days she admittedly prefers daily routines and repetitive rituals that stabilize her life within, what she calls, "the comfort of the expected."

The Queen could have told her that. Her enduring popularity is largely based, like a lifelong friend, on the chummy warmth of predictability. To most of her subjects, Elizabeth's yearly routines, her ability to avoid scandal, even her hairdo has been the one constant in their lives. While her bearskin-capped sentries shuffle about daily, she is, in a real sense, the one unchanging guard of Britain. "She has been there all my life," said actress Dame Maggie Smith (of *Downton Abbey* fame). "I can't imagine her not being there. I just can't." On her Golden Jubilee, Prince Charles got the whole country nodding when he rightly called his mother "a beacon of tradition and stability in the midst of profound, sometimes perilous change." Adjectives like "dependable," "reliable," "steady" and "stable" trip lightly from the tongue of anyone who has spent any length of time with the Queen, including her most hardened critics. Helen Mirren may have begun her role in *The Queen* with borderline disdain for the Crown, but she finished filled with deep respect for the woman who wears it. "To be that consistent for that long is amazingly comforting," said Mirren. "It shows such reliability. She has never lurched in one direction or another."

*

Like Mirren, we're all drawn to the predictable because our brains simply work better that way. Whether you call them routines, habits or daily rituals, acts of repetition are crucial for higher levels of thinking. Routines set our bodies on cruise control, the easiest route between us and the majority of life's tasks, freeing our brains to concentrate on higher matters above the mundane (e.g., you can theoretically compose a sonnet while brushing your teeth). And though we often confuse the mindlessness of routines with limiting the flow of our mental juices, it's actually the reverse. The more you ground your day in routines, the more brainpower you have left over for bigger problems. In a study of workers at a high-tech German company, sociologists found that employees who embraced the highest levels of "routinization" in their job were more, not less, likely to come up with new ideas and product improvements than their more free-styling coworkers. The repetitive working patterns of history's best-known artists, novelists and philosophers reveal the same.* As Scott Adams, creator of the *Dilbert* comic strip, explains, his mornings are purposefully built on repeated regimens, "step for step, every day" even down to his ritualized protein bar for breakfast. "In other words," he says, "I set my personal body on autopilot for the morning. That frees my brain for creativity." This alone might explain why children, with their higher outputs of imagination, thrive under the security of routines (and go wacko when their eating and sleeping schedules aren't stable). Years ago, when Lady Bonham-Carter's son paid a visit to Elizabeth and Margaret at Windsor Castle during World War II, exchanging a life of wartime uncertainties for a regimen of royal order, the Queen Mother recorded the almost overnight changes in their young visitor's demeanor. "I am so glad to know that the respectable routine at Windsor has rested and restored him," she wrote. "There is a 'governess and schoolroom' atmosphere there at the moment which . . . is very healing!"

Royal routines tend to take on a "serenely" religious quality, says British historian David Starkey, who describes the Queen's working life as "more of a liturgy than a diary" of random dates and engagements. A life which is soothingly cyclical, "like the Church's liturgical year, which it so much resembled," he says. This may not be surprising for someone who, like Elizabeth, has been all-out "anointed" by the Archbishop of Canterbury. Religious communities throughout western Europe have for centuries relied on the clarity and focus only routines can bring. But others less ecclesiastically endowed have found that tapping into the same tradition can have dramatic effects. Inspired by the strict schedules of monastic life (practiced by clear-thinkers like Mother Teresa), writer Holly Pierlot abandoned her freewheeling working style and put herself on a modified "rule of life"—a daily plan with an allocated time frame for every priority, even play and rest. Prior to the experiment, what she

---

* See Mason Currey's extensive profiles of famous working habits in *Daily Rituals: How Artists Work*.

thought would crush her "cherished spontaneity" turned out to be life-changing. Writing in *A Mother's Rule of Life*, Pierlot discovered that tightly focused schedules "freed my mind from a thousand cares and concerns. Whereas before I would stare around the house, wondering which task to tackle first, and as I worked on one, a hundred new ones would come in to worry me, now I knew exactly when every task in my home was going to be done. Knowing that tidy-up came just before supper made me stop tidying up constantly throughout the day." Pierlot argued, "My cherished spontaneity was pointless when I didn't have the time or energy to enjoy it."

The Queen's own daily schedule, which she calls her "timetable," serves an identical purpose. It not only focuses her concentration on the task at hand—be it a red box or rendezvous with the prime minster—it sets important limits on those obligations, allocating time for other personal priorities, like breaks and breathers throughout the day, moments Elizabeth would likely never find time for without.* As psychologists are now well aware, written goals and schedules work so well in this regard because they help us avoid the all-too common "Zeigarnik effect." This is your brain's uncanny (and obnoxious) ability to nag you about obligations in life either left undone or ominously upcoming. The Zeigarnik effect is what turns minds into leaky faucets of persistent to-do lists; and it's one of the top culprits of workplace distractions today. As Holly Pierlot observed, to begin one task is only to release a floodgate of "a hundred new ones" to worry out, all vying for equal attention. Writing down specific plans for tackling each job, however, has been shown to be an effective antidote to this looping brain quirk. It's as if your subconscious mind *wants* you to create a mental framework on which to place and prioritize each unfinished task, and will allow you to work uninterrupted only once you do so. This accounts for the workplace distinction visible across a wide range of professions: people who write down goals are substantially more likely to accomplish

---

* The Queen's timetable can be incredibly tight, sometimes down to the minute. Biographer Sarah Bradford recounts one evening near the beginning of her reign when Elizabeth met with the president of France at 6:30 p.m., the president of Turkey at 6:45 p.m. and the president of the Praesidium of Yugoslavia at 7:00 p.m.

them, methodically ticking each task off, one at a time.

*

The whole point and purpose of the Queen's timetable is to be limiting, to remind her of her own physical limits. The result, ironically, has given her more freedom and flexibility, not less, in her life's work. The English essayist G. K. Chesterton brilliantly explained the positive paradox of limitations in this way: Imagine a playground positioned near a dangerous cliff. A high fence skirts its edges, protecting the children inside, who run free and wild within its secure boundaries. Now imagine the fence was removed. The children immediately stop running and jumping about, and soon stop doing much of anything at all, save huddling together in a mass of uncertainty far away from the precipice. To Chesterton, absolute freedom involved knowing where to put the fence on your personal frontiers. Boundless joy was found in "the liberty to bind myself," he believed. Almost an exact echo of the ancient wisdom psychologist Mihaly Csikszentmihalyi imparts in his classic treatise on achieving optimal life experiences: "Cicero once wrote that to be completely free one must become a slave to a set of laws. In other words, accepting limitations is liberating." Royal rituals have taught Elizabeth when to say yes to new demands on her time and, more importantly, when to say no. Pity Prince Charles didn't pick up the habit sooner. He spent most of his adult life running himself, his staff and his wife Diana ragged by his all-out rebellion of predictable routines and personal limits. "I tend to lead a sort of idiotic existence," he once admitted during a television interview. "[I'm] trying to get involved in too many things and dashing about. This is going to be my problem— trying to sort of control myself." In the memorable words of one Palace aide, getting Charles to stick to any well-defined program "was like nailing jellies to a wall."

Wisdom often skips a generation, especially among royalty. Prince William is far more like his grandmother when it comes to appreciating the Most Excellent Order of *order* itself. During his early education at Eton, William flourished under the school's famously structured regime, far removed from the tumultuous family drama he once experienced at home. Much like the Queen's timetable, William's days at Eton were tightly packed with more activities and commitments (stretching from 7:30 a.m. to 10:00 p.m.) than most adults experience in a week. Yet they all existed within a logical routine that became not only familiar and healing for the traumatized prince but also positively preparative. William is now immensely more adept at balancing the tricky triune demands of royal heir, husband and dad than his own troubled father ever was.

Today a "Norland" nanny is now firmly established in William and Kate's nursery, helping to raise the next generation of royals. Graduates of the prestigious Norland College, Norland nannies are known for their stalwart beliefs in consistency and order. Its most famous alumni, Brenda Ashford, was one of Britain's longest-serving and most beloved nannies. With a career spanning 62 years caring for countless children, her nurseries were such successful incubators of love and discipline, families continued to beg for Ashford's services well into her eighties. Often asked what her secret was, she responded with timeworn certainty, "It's simple really. All babies thrive on routine." Apparently none of us grow out of it. Not even the Queen of England, who still works best by listening to her inner nanny.*

---

* And up until the early 1990s, listening to her real one too. Nanny "Bobo" never left the Queen's side for 67 years. Seamlessly morphing into Elizabeth's official "dresser" in adulthood, Bobo became her lifelong confidant, one of the few unbroken links to her childhood, and was reportedly the only person, outside the family, allowed to call the Queen by her childhood nickname, "Lilibet."

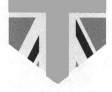

THE BUCKINGHAM SYSTEM

OR RULE #6—SURVIVAL OF THE COURTEOUS

Beware! You are entering an old-fashioned establishment.
—SIGNPOST OUTSIDE A ROYAL RESIDENCE

U nder the usual standards of *workplace behaviors likely to occasion a heart attack*, the Queen shouldn't even be alive. At the very least, she should be a haggard, stress-oozing executive working herself to a spastic end. A cardiac time bomb for Crown and country, as it were. It should be the textbook fate of anyone who's on the job 24/7, working every day of the calendar year, save Christmas and Easter. Someone whose evenings and weekends are often not her own, but spent in hundreds of various job-related events at home and throughout the world. Someone who, either by choice or parliamentary coercion, emits definite whiffs of a type A workaholic. "I must go do my boxes," the Queen once said while staying with friends. "Oh must you ma'am?" the group implored. "If I missed one once, I would never get it straight again," the Queen replied.

To royal biographers, this grind is simply the "occupational hazard" of kingship, a professional burden that should have killed Elizabeth years ago. And for your typical CEO, it might well have. But Buckingham Palace isn't your typical corporation. Demonstrating an almost organic survival mechanism, the monarchy has evolved and adapted itself to accommodate the demanding pressures placed on its sovereign. Over time, it has grown a protective cocoon designed to reduce the stress that has crippled past kings. You could call it *The Buckingham System*. And for royals like Elizabeth who continue to institute its rules, accomplishing a Queen-sized to-do list can be just another pleasant day at the office.

Accustomed to the frenzied, cutthroat pace of their own office cultures, journalists who enter Buckingham Palace are often dazzled by the palpable difference—namely, a pervading sense of calm. Once through its doors, a sort of time travel occurs, says royal chronicler Brian Hoey, back to a bygone era "of quiet tranquility." Even the staff talk in chivalrous overtones, regardless of the situation. Take the marvelous example recounted by author Basil Boothroyd. During one of his visits to the Palace, gathering research for a biography on Prince Philip, Boothroyd had a chance encounter with the Queen's private secretary, Michael Adeane, as he was crossing the forecourt at a quick pace. Adeane halted immediately, extended the politest greeting, exchanged pleasantries about the weather and kindly inquired about the progress of Boothroyd's book. Having thoroughly showered Boothroyd with courtesy, Adeane softly added, almost as an aside, "If you'll forgive me, I must be on my way now. I've just heard that my house is on fire. I wouldn't mind, but as it's part of St. James's Palace . . ."

Similar tales of workplace civility emerged from the Queen Mother's household—like the crash course in workplace civility Major Colin Burgess received when he became the Queen Mother's equerry in 1994. Fresh from the army and accustomed to issuing the odd brusque order, Burgess was dumbfounded by his inability to get the staff to follow his simplest commands. "My initial intuition was to treat the lower orders as subordinates and address them as such," he admitted. He would fire off a quick order to the Queen Mother's chauffeur, only to hear the curt response, "Well, not if you ask me like that." Finally an older and wiser employee taught him the ropes of respectful royal service. Turns out Burgess was a bit too prickly around the edges, and as soon as he turned his orders into gentle requests, peppering them with ample p's and q's, as if he were asking a favor "in a very nice kind of conversational way," the staff were happy to oblige. "[I thought] the whole place was utterly mad," says Burgess.

Then again, these protocols of courtesy come straight from the top. The Queen is "extraordinarily respectful of other people," says Mark Greene, who wrote a book on Elizabeth's behind-the-scenes character. She has never referred to her employees as "servants" and sees it as a mark of genuine disrespect to make anyone wait for her, however lofty or lowly their position. Moreover, the rare moments in which she has displayed the merest wobble of an angry outburst can be counted on one hand.* It's a top-down culture of respect that strongly influenced the famously calm demeanor of one of her favorite private secretaries, Martin Charteris. Though he dealt with frequent attacks from an increasingly vicious press, Charteris is said to have lived by the Palace-inspired doctrine: "Everybody I meet I vow only one thing, to be relentlessly agreeable to them." The Queen has had to entertain brutal dictators, pompous presidents and untold number of celebrities she isn't particularly enamored with, yet polite respect has been her MO for every one of them. When French president Jacques Chirac spent an evening at Windsor Castle in 2004, the sumptuously appointed Waterloo Chamber in which he was entertained was temporarily renamed "the Music Room," as the Queen felt that sitting in a chamber dedicated to Britain's decisive victory over Napoleon's army wouldn't be altogether comfortable for the head of France. Elizabeth believes that such small niceties matter. And so they do in unexpectedly big ways. Though you'll have to look further afield than Windsor to find the evidence.

The business culture of Japan, for instance, is built on the same courteous standards. Politeness is so endemic among Japanese workers,

---

* Most are infinitesimally brief, but entertaining. Take Elizabeth's rather sensible reply to photographer Annie Leibovitz who wanted to capture the Queen in formal Garter robe and tiara for a photo shoot in 2007. After Elizabeth spent considerable time in her dressing room complying with the request, Leibovitz had an artsy change of mind—perhaps Her Majesty could remove the "crown" to appear less dressy. "Less dressy!" said Elizabeth, pointing to her voluminous velvet Garter robe, "What do you think this is?" The culture historian Peter Conrad makes a good point: "Imagine the Statue of Liberty's reaction if a stylist had said, 'Honey, let's lose the torch.'"

translating Western concepts such as "competition," "aggression" and "assertiveness" into the language is almost impossible. Even casually referring to your coworker by his or her first name could be crossing the line of rudeness in Japan. With all this interpersonal care and consideration going around, the fact that Japan boasts enviously low rates of heart disease may not come as a great surprise. And yet, when you consider the Japanese relentless work ethic, their penchant for long hours at the office, for taking little vacation time and for creating some of the wonkiest workaholics in the developed world, it starts getting confusing. Social psychologist Robert Levine believes the answer lies in Japan's unique workplace atmosphere. Whereas forceful competition and hostility can get you ahead in America, it can also create corporate cultures of stress that contribute to our high rates of heart disease. In Japan, type A workers are unquestionably valued, but "hostility and anger . . . play little part in the hardworking, fast pace of the Japanese," says Levine. Suggesting that "as long as work is approached with the right attitude—without hostility or competitiveness—there appears to be little or no increased risk for coronary heart disease," he says.*

*

Back at the Palace, maintaining corporate tranquility is business as usual. Few can forget the scolding Italian politician Silvio Berlusconi received when he kept disrespectfully raising his voice at the G20 summit in 2009. After a particularly earsplitting shout across the room, the Queen had heard quite enough. "What is it?" she asked the assembled world leaders. "Why does he have to shout?" However critical the situation, loudmouthed hysterics has never been the appropriate response in royal circles. Years ago, American ambassador Joseph Kennedy witnessed it firsthand while taking tea at the Palace with George VI and his wife. All was proceeding smoothly until Elizabeth's aunt, elderly Lady Elphinstone, started displaying the symptoms of a heart attack. Expecting everyone to launch into the screaming abdabs, Kennedy watched in

---

* Interestingly, as more American-inspired corporate attitudes (like high-pressure competition) invade traditional Japanese workplaces, its people are now being warned of an entirely new cultural conception: *karoshi*, "death from overwork."

amazement as those around him "retained [their] composure." Medical assistance was summoned, and Kennedy was assured that he need not slink away in awkwardness or terror, indeed that "Lady Elphinstone was [feeling] better."

A peaceful office culture is the residual perk of being part of a centuries-old institution that has seen it *all* before, one that knows how it will calmly handle every eventuality. As a Palace insider explained, if a foreign enemy landed on the shores of England today, the Queen would simply stop what she was doing and calmly say, "I must let the Lord Lieutenant know." Because whatever workplace stress the Queen might experience in her job, the stress of "what if" is not one of them. Elizabeth and her staff are master forecasters, planning years in advance for the best- and worst-case scenarios, all under the anxiety-reducing premise that "any crisis could be handled, as long as proper procedures were followed," according to biographer Carolly Erickson. The unexpected death of Princess Diana in a Parisian hospital in 1997 might have sent the media into a frenzy of unknowns, but the Palace already had a plan in place for the death of any royal who dies overseas and needs to be sent back to England for burial. Code name "Operation Overlord" was thus calmly set in motion, allowing Elizabeth time to concentrate on cherishing her grandsons through the tragedy.

Hence the wonderful paradox to all this forward thinking, it enables the Queen to live in the present, to literally achieve the "presence of mind" she is famous for. In other words, Elizabeth isn't a fan of the modern mayhem known as multitasking. She might juggle more job titles than any other person on earth (from Lord High Admiral of the Royal Navy to Paramount Chief of Fiji) but "at her desk she is a marvel of concentration and accuracy" says Elizabeth Longford, one of the many biographers to notice the Queen's "methodical manner of going about things." Like the sugar crystals of her childhood, Elizabeth lines up each day's obligations and tackles them individually, with dogged concentration. Remarkably, almost a hundred years ago, *The Times* predicted exactly that, that a monarch's success wouldn't depend on their ability to multitask, nor their "intellectual brilliance . . . but upon the moral qualities of steadiness [and] staying-power"—a statement which could extend to virtually any profession today.

Granted, multitasking might not be immoral, but it isn't the divine skill of the highly productive either. In fact, its very existence is turning out to be a modern myth altogether. As the latest research shows, our bodies might be able to perform more than one mindless task at a time, as a circus clown might eat a cake while balancing another on his bottom, but our brains are downright delinquent when it comes to *focusing* on two things at once (consider the outrageous number of accidents caused by people who think they can text and drive simultaneously—or walk while talking on their phones, without bumping into an adjacent light post). Stanford professor Clifford Nass was one of the first to debunk the myth. Pitching self-described "multitaskers" against their single-tasking peers in a variety of problem-solving tests, Nass found something so contrary to popular expectations, "It keeps me up late at night," he admits. Multitaskers not only demonstrated that they were more easily distracted than single-taskers, they were outperformed on every measure of accuracy, speed, organization and the ability to filter out irrelevant data. "Multitaskers were just lousy at everything," concluded Nass.

Even the word "multitasking" is technically a misnomer. Since true mental focus is limited to single tasks, people who mince about with giant macchiatos in hand, thinking they are multitasking throughout the day, are actually doing what researchers call "task switching"—leaping back and forth between tasks as quickly as possible. But there's nothing particularly zippy about task switching. Every time you bounce from one job to another, your brain needs time to recover, to essentially reacquaint itself with the ground rules of that particular job and pick up where it left off. This can take a few seconds or a few minutes, depending on the complexity of the task—piffling figures, perhaps, but repeat them often enough and these recovery times will add up enormously. Researches now estimate that workers lose almost a third of their day simply recovering from the distractions of our task-switching culture.

＊

Focus fatigue is nothing new. Back in the reign of George V, Queen Mary complained about the niggling distractions and "hourly interruptions" that beset her and the King at work. "There is nothing more fatiguing &

quite wears one out," she said. "It is far less tiring to work at one thing for three hours than to have to turn one's thoughts to different subjects every few minutes, jumping from an important subject, to some minor one, & vice versa, oh! I know it well." What Queen Mary would make of our modern cacophony of attention-grabbing texts, tweets, dings, rings and posts is a sobering thought. And it probably explains one of the wisest workplace decisions Elizabeth has ever made: her refusal to be tethered to a cell phone. Prince Andrew technically gave her one in 2001, and her grandsons have long since taught her how to text,* but she has never been spotted messing with the digital doohickey either at work or in public. Elizabeth might have graciously accepted the iPod President Obama presented her with in 2007, but she doesn't like what the gadgets are doing to her subjects. "I miss seeing their eyes," she touchingly told US ambassador Matthew Barzun, regretting the strange way electronic screens and camera phones now come between her and the faces of her adoring crowds. To quote Princess Anne, someone slightly more blunt, the public's trust in the questionable *smartness* of smartphones is just plain "weird."

It's a fair charge against devices that are purposefully designed to be more addictive than they are assistive. According to former Google employee Tristan Harris, smartphone algorithms share intentional similarities to slot machines, one of the most compulsively addictive inventions in human history. In their whirling, buzzing, attention-grabbing pings of messages and posts, smartphones create loops of unpredictable anticipation that keep us coming back for more and more. Americans check their phones an average of 52 times a day, making unintended screen "time" the leading hijacker of our own precious time. As the Duchess of York discovered, once attempting to keep up with this new onslaught of data and messages, "modern modes of communication" can turn us into "the sorcerer's apprentice at war with too many mops," sweeping up too many self-generating puddles. "By saving time with technology," she realized, "I'd lost half my day!"

---

* Prankster Prince Harry reportedly used the opportunity to record the following voice mail message on his grandmother's cell: "Hey, wassup? This is Liz! Sorry I'm away from the throne. For a hotline to Philip, press one; for Charles, press two; for the corgis, press three."

Aside from strict necessities, cell phones were all but banned at the Palace until fairly recently, and Elizabeth might still chill you to the core if one goes off inappropriately in her presence. Like the time Clare Short, the overseas development secretary, failed to silence her mobile during a high-level meeting with the Queen. When it chanced to go off, Elizabeth didn't miss a beat. "Do answer it, dear," she said. "It might be somebody important."

On the surface, it's an odd stance for a type A go-getter like Elizabeth, who can accomplish more in one week than some people do in an entire year and exclaim, at the end of it, with all sincerity, "I am an amazing woman!" But in choosing not to keep up with the technological Joneses, the Queen is actually making her amazing accomplishments possible.* Because at one of the oldest continuous-operating office building in London, speed doesn't always equal success, if sanity, stress and human courtesy is sacrificed. After all, some messages are still best digested when delivered the royally old-fashioned way: at a walking pace on a silver platter.

---

* Anyone who wishes to follow suit should consult the tremendously helpful *How to Break Up with Your Phone* by Catherine Price. A small decision like turning off email notifications alone can greatly improve the productivity of your day.

AIRS AND GRACES

OR RULE #7—NEVER SLOUCH
IN YOUR OWN PRESENCE

Poise is Power.

—FLORENCE SCOVEL SHINN

The overwhelming presence of greatness being what it is, you'd expect a face-to-face encounter with the Queen to go in a physically downward direction. Namely, it would turn most people into jelly-backed genuflectors attempting their deepest bow or curtsey (with points awarded for head-to-floor contact, similar to a sycophantic extra in *The King and I*). Rather fantastically, it causes the reverse. People who meet the Queen for the first time instinctively stand taller, straighter and more skeletally vertical than they have in years. "She's a stiffener of backs," admitted Martin Charteris, recounting the thousands of slumped spines that have been miraculously straightened in her presence.* Politicians and celebrities can hardly visit the Palace without body language experts suggesting countless theories for their newfound poise. But there's a simpler explanation. Like the monarchial version of monkey see, monkey do, everyone is simply aping the standards of the most physically upright sovereign alive.

---

* With the famous exception of Margaret Thatcher, known for dropping such preposterously low curtseys, they tended to make the Queen feel uncomfortable. "Her curtsey almost reached Australia," said Lord Powell, one of Thatcher's principal aides.

To listen to royal biographers, Elizabeth's posture is something of a national treasure. It's easy to see why. A steady head on steady shoulders guiding a steady monarchy makes for great royal symbolism. There's always been a certain cachet for those who can strike a regally straight pose, and it certainly helped Elizabeth at the start of her career. For many of her subjects, it was visual proof of her natural right to reign.* Her first prime minister, Winston Churchill, being among them. Before he became acquainted with her deeper qualities, Churchill was relieved that, at the very least, Elizabeth *looked* like a Queen. "All the film people in the world, if they had scoured the globe, could not have found anyone so suited to the part," he said. Inspired by visions of a new Elizabethan age, other onlookers praised the Queen's poise with more courtly language. Lady Airlie, for one, was positively smitten by the noble "carriage of her head" (i.e., it didn't lunge forward like a country bumpkin). Others liked to quote the poet Alexander Pope, "What winning graces! What majestic mien! She moves a Goddess, and she looks a queen!" This sort of hyperbole has quieted down over the years, as Elizabeth has ranked in grander accomplishments above that of a standard twelve-inch ruler. But all things considered, her legacy of excellent posture remains justifiably impressive.

According to biographer Ingrid Seward, someone who has tracked the Queen's every move for decades, Elizabeth has never once slouched on the throne, or any chair for that matter. Writing in 2015, Seward reports, "in all her seventy-seven years [in the public eye] the Queen had always sat straight . . . during even the dullest of speeches." Those who have observed her even more closely—photographers and artists, for instance—say the same. Australian painter William Dargie once spent seven long sessions with the Queen capturing her likeness for a commemorative portrait and walked away stunned at the fact that her "straight back . . . never slumped once." Like most women of her generation and class, Elizabeth picked up the postural habit very early in life,

---

* This isn't as far-fetched as it sounds. In the 1920s, when one "Anna Anderson" claimed to be the long-lost Grand Duchess Anastasia, youngest daughter of the last Russian tsar, her supporters argued the case based on little more than the serene quality of her excellent posture, claiming such natural deportment could only have been acquired in a courtly environment.

and probably for little more than displays of "good breeding," at first. The Queen Mother was always adamant that "a lady's back should never touch the back of her chair." And yet the habit has gone on to have far more tangible benefits to Elizabeth's daily work.

*

It's hardly what you'd expect from the most prestigious job in Britain, but clerical paper-pushing makes up a large portion of the Queen's day. Those red boxes piled with governmental papers can pin her to a desk for hours on end. So as occupational statistics go, Elizabeth *should* be ravaged by the same scourge affecting deskbound workers worldwide—specifically lower back, neck, shoulder, chest and hip pain. Sedentary tasks are becoming such an oddly hazardous business, seated office workers now find themselves at higher risks for incurring musculoskeletal injuries than workers in any other industry sector, including (and here the mind boggles) the construction industry. Yet Elizabeth has sailed through these deskbound perils relatively unscathed. "There was no such thing as backache" in the Queen's long career, says biographer Elizabeth Longford. And her gracefully erect spine has had much to do with that.

Clarissa Eden, wife of Prime Minister Anthony Eden, once watched Elizabeth at work and noted how properly she would "sit up at a slight distance from the chair back" while keeping her own back perfectly straight. "She can sit like that for hours," marveled Eden. This might sound exhaustingly painful for the unpracticed, but maintaining good posture while sitting is the only way to avoid chronic muscular and skeletal pain in the long run. Elizabeth's straight-back technique, moreover, happens to be the same graceful pose recommended by physical therapists as the easiest and cheapest antidote for office-related aches.* The most expensive ergonomic chair doesn't come close to matching the pain-free support your body can provide naturally.

---

* To sit more like a queen, pain-free living expert Lee Albert recommends starting with the postural version of training wheels. Get a small, malleable pillow—the cheaper the better, he says. Sit up straight in the chair, roll or scrunch the pillow and wedge it tightly in the gap between the chair and your lower back. Adjust the pillow's support thickness until your head is positioned directly over your shoulders.

Good posture has always felt naturally comfortable to Elizabeth, even from a young age. There's an iconic photograph of her as a princess in the late 1930s: She's out camping on the Frogmore estate, standing alongside a troop of Girl Guides beside a giant tree. Yet while the other girls in the picture are absentmindedly relaxed, loose limbed and slouching, Elizabeth (little more than eleven) is standing perfectly straight. No doubt you would too if you had Queen Mary for a grandmother, someone believed to be largely responsible for forming Elizabeth's early poise. Standing famously firm herself, Queen Mary could appear inches taller than her husband the King (which she wasn't), thanks to the formidable straightness of her "magnificent carriage," as it was called. Elizabeth would be molded in her image. "Teach that child not to fidget," she instructed the royal nannies. Early photographs show how quickly the lesson was learned. In a 1932 snapshot Elizabeth can be spotted riding in an open-air carriage with her grandparents, smiling and remaining remarkably upright for a six-year-old. To observers, even to the Queen Mother herself, Elizabeth seemed to practically emerge from the womb sitting "bolt upright."

But Queen Mary can't take all the credit. In all probability, you popped into the world with the same posture reflex too. All healthy babies do. As soon as they're able to sit independently, babies quickly find their center of gravity and instinctively support themselves with near perfect spinal alignment. Toddlers likewise walk with straighter backs than most runway models, thanks to their intuitive compliance with the body's preferred mode of balance: weight evenly distributed on both legs with the head in its most stable position directly over the shoulders. But through a host of bad habits, mostly picked up at school, hunched over a desk, most of us lose our innate sense of physical equilibrium. The posture instinct is still there, however. You're reminded of it (usually through an ache) every time you sit or stand improperly for prolonged periods of time. The body simply needs to relearn how this natural alignment feels.*

---

* For starters, try what I call "the Claire-Foy Technique," after the actress who stands with impeccably good posture in *The Crown*, season one and two. Keeping your hands royally cupped in front of your stomach, like Claire, serves as a makeshift back brace, not only

Having a persistent granny paid off for Elizabeth here. She was never allowed to outgrow what should feel most natural for everyone. Though the Queen realizes she's somewhat of an anomaly in this regard and has willingly offered pointers to those who have misplaced their own posture mechanism. Susan Crosland, wife of the Queen's foreign secretary, received one of these impromptu lessons in the 1970s, after looking mystified at the way Elizabeth could stand for hours at diplomatic events without tiring. "One plants one's feet apart like this," explained the Queen, lifting her gown above her ankles in demonstration. "Always keep them parallel. Make sure your weight is evenly distributed. That's all there is to it."

And there you have the instantly recognizable "Windsor stance," which Helen Mirren perfected so well in her role in *The Queen*. It's a stance which has prevented untold number of royally sore feet, for sure, but has also promoted a great deal of physical stability too. Years of practicing good posture has had a bracing effect on the Queen's sense of balance. Well into the danger years of elderly wobbles, when many people her age are suffering crippling falls, Elizabeth has kept her inner gyroscope remarkably well calibrated. What could have been a potentially disastrous incident in 2013 proved it. At 87 years old, the Queen was inspecting renovations at her Sandringham estate when she entered a darkened outbuilding and tripped over the threshold. Quickly moving to catch her, architect Charles Morris was amazed to find his rescue attempt unnecessary. The Queen instantly regained balance and righted herself naturally.* Royal biographers can wax poetic about how this inner stability has played out on a larger scale, righting the monarchy through its own wobbling years of uncertainty, but there's more than a scientific grain of truth behind the idea. Adopting regally good posture

---

reminding you to stand tall, but providing some helpful support in the process. Speaking of support, the Queen isn't opposed to using a corrective shoulder pad, under her clothes, to help round out her posture, especially as she has aged.

* Incidents like this have reinforced the wisdom of the Queen's "heel height" stipulation. When it comes to shoes, she is inflexibly sensible. Elizabeth "will not entertain a heel higher than 2.25 inches," says British fashion expert Sali Hughes.

has not only made Elizabeth *look* more like a confident queen, it has, in all likelihood, made her *feel* more like one too.

※

Arguably the most fascinating discoveries in applied psychology in recent years have focused on posture's ability to affect people's mood. What British fiction writer Muriel Spark merely hinted at in 1963—that good posture is "an equanimity of body and mind . . . [contributing] to the attainment of self-confidence"—now has factual support. There are neurological chain reactions just waiting to be released when we stretch ourselves into our most upright position. Hormones like testosterone (giving us feelings of power and competence), serotonin (regulating our mood and happiness) and cortisol (controlling stress) are all dramatically affected by our physical poise. Posture is so powerful, recovering alcoholics who adopt better posture are less likely to relapse than those who slouch, inadvertently adopting the posture of weakness and defeat. The same goes for people who struggle with depression, anxiety, risk aversion or simply low energy levels—all can benefit, remarkably, by simply standing or sitting up straight. Every time we expand our outward self—standing taller, stretching our shoulders back—our inner being is simultaneously strengthened, potentially starting "a psychological cascade that lasts all day," says social psychologist Dana Carney. Moods are lifted, energy levels rise and a cocktail of confidence-boosting neurochemicals are released, compelling you to stand taller still. "And—boom—a positive cycle begins," adds Carney.*

From a royal perspective, a piece of near identical wisdom was recently offered by His Serene Highness Alexi Lubomirski in his book *Princely Advice for a Happy Life*. Long since bereft of his family's princely throne in Poland (and currently working as a photographer),

---

* Good posture can even trigger self-control. In a 1999 study, researchers set out to discover whether they could increase the willpower of college students, assigning them a variety of self-control exercises to practice for a couple of weeks (from maintaining better moods to practicing better posture). Unexpectedly, the students who simply reminded themselves to sit and stand up straighter for a couple of weeks showed the highest overall improvements in willpower.

Lubomirski sought to instruct his children on how to conduct themselves like royalty without enjoying any of its palatial trappings. And posture, he believes, is essential to this end:

> Your posture can define your mood. Sit up straight and strong. This will allow energy to flow more freely in your body. . . . When you walk, walk tall. Breathe deeply. Feel your chest expand and smile with your whole body at the blessing of life. Let people see a proud, confident, strong, and happy spirit.

Elizabeth would certainly relate. As would everyone who, by her upright example, has felt themselves becoming "bigger, prouder, bolder and more heroic" in her presence, says journalist John Walsh. Slumping is so *lèse-majesté*, an offense against the dignity of monarchy, it's proactively mentioned up front, in the seven-page document handed out to entertainers before performing at the Palace. Whatever celebrity you boast, there will be absolutely no slouching or leaning against bars or tables whilst in the Queen's company. Those who remember the rule go further at the Palace. Those who don't, well, you can attach your own meaning to British playwright Alan Bennett's pronouncement: "Subjects seldom sulked to the Queen, as they were not entitled to, and once upon a time it would have taken them to the Tower."

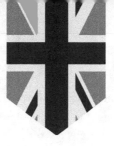

VIVE LE DEVOIR

OR RULE #8—REAL QUEENS DON'T RETIRE

I will remain on the throne until I fall off.
—MARGRETHE II, QUEEN OF DENMARK

In 2002 the Archbishop of Canterbury, George Carey, dropped by the Palace to convey an important message to the Queen. At age 66 and already a full year past Britain's mandatory retirement age, the time had come, he said, to hand the bishop's staff on to someone younger and altogether more springy than himself. There must have been a wistful look in the Archbishop's eye which seemed to say *won't you consider joining me, ma'am?* because the Queen replied in all frankness, "Oh, that's something I can't do. I am going to carry on to the end." If this didn't make Carey feel like an infantile underachiever (Elizabeth was pushing 76 at the time), it certainly raised some well-meant questions and concerns throughout the country. Considering her decades of dutiful service, why *can't* the Queen rest on her royal laurels and call it a job well done, passing the scepter on to her next heir (by which the public usually means conveniently bypassing Charles and crowning William instead)? Monarchs throughout Europe, far younger than Elizabeth, are quite merrily dropping off their thrones like flies. Queen Beatrix of the Netherlands, King Juan Carlos of Spain and King Albert II of the Belgians have all decided to call it quits in recent years, putting their more youthful progenies in charge. Even Pope Benedict

XVI guiltlessly rode the "resignation" wave in 2013, exchanging St. Peter's throne for a quiet life in the country. Surely Elizabeth has earned the right too. Perhaps it might even add a few more years to her already long life. But retirement isn't always the cure-all it's cracked up to be, and separating a person from their life's work can be fraught with unintended consequences. As one Palace courtier reminded the public, "We have beheaded monarchs, usurped monarchs, but we do not have retired monarchs." There are very good reasons for that.

For starters, it has nothing to do with stubborn tenacity. Elizabeth II is not mimicking her Elizabethan forebearer, an elderly tyrant refusing to share authority and clutching her crown for dear life. The Crown *is* Elizabeth II's life: a twofer package with inseparable symbiosis of duty and identity. As she is wont to point out to anyone who casually drops the hint of abdication, "In this existence, the job and the life go together. You can't really divide it up." According to Andrew Marr, Elizabeth belongs to a generation who took pride in defining themselves by their work (be they farmer, shoemaker or sovereign)—a role that didn't automatically stop just because somebody reached some magical number in their sixties. Queen Mary was positively flummoxed when she heard that Queen Wilhelmina of the Netherlands was abdicating in favor of her daughter in 1948: "Wilhelmina is only sixty-eight and that is *no* age to give up your job." Nothing good could come out of it, she thought, and quite rightly too.

It's long been observed that people whose work entails a high sense of responsibility and social contribution (policemen and teachers, for example) don't fare so well after retirement. To lose their role is to lose a large chunk of themselves along with it, and a staggering number experience declines in their health shortly after retirement, including their mental health. Retirees soon experience a 40 percent increase in their risk of developing depression and a 60 percent uptick in their probability of developing at least one diagnosed physical ailment. This explains why traditional cultures define the "good life"—even in old age—in very different terms. Rather than viewing retirement as one long hammock swing with Jimmy Buffett's "Margaritaville" looping in the background, a life completely devoid of meaningful work has never been our collective instinct for self-preservation. The long-lived Japanese don't even have a comparable word for "retire" in their language, not in the Western sense of a complete break between their jobs and themselves. If they leave a company, people in Japan retain a very fluid concept of their personal working talents, finding ways to carry over their skills and crafts into old age. The notion of *taking it easy* is as little discussed among the Japanese as it is at Buckingham Palace. Instead, they remain painters and woodcutters and pearl divers as long as their health allows.* Their guiding principal being an intuitive concept they call *ikigai*—the polar opposite of laid-back retirement, sometimes loosely translated as "the happiness of always being busy."

A longtime admirer of Eastern wisdom, Prince Charles is plainly acquainted with the concept. On a recent trip to Malta, Charles was touring the city of Mdina when he spotted an elderly shopkeeper who he remembered meeting on his first trip to the island in 1968. "I'm ninety-one," boasted the agile shopkeeper. "You're not!" replied Charles. "I'm nearly seventy!" Then he added, as if he was imparting an esoteric secret of longevity, "Keep working! Don't ever stop." The irony is, the longer Charles's mother abides by the same secret, the less likely he will inherit the throne anytime soon.

The late Queen Mother saw to that. She raised Elizabeth to have a strong sense of personal *devoir*, a more genteel word for "duty"—literally that which you owe yourself and the world around you. If any member of the family was shirking his or her responsibilities, the Queen Mother only needed to whisper the word for the culprit to quickly get the message. One never abandons one's "devoir." And you certainly don't retire from it. "It's no good sitting back," the Queen Mother would say, when "your *devoir*, your duty" compels you on.

＊

---

* If you enjoy your job, maintaining a low level of occupational stress is actually good for you. Dr. Howard S. Friedman, professor of psychology at the University of California, Riverside, spent more than twenty years following a group of test subjects and discovered that people who kept working with sustained dedication to their job, despite its challenges, lived longer than people who opted for early retirement and a pressure-free lifestyle.

We find an almost exact parallel in the ancient Greek concept of *eudaimonia*. Coined and popularized by Aristotle, it advanced the idea that everyone had a divine spark within them, a true self, which marked each person out for a unique calling or destiny. Practically every school of ancient philosophy agreed that the "good life" was impossible without following one's inner eudaimonic compass which, more often than not, points to bigger and better things. Children seem to recognize this intuitively. The least egotistical child will often harbor secret suspicions that they are somehow special and uniquely set apart from the crowd. Raised on fairy tales and imaginary kingdoms, these tend to involve a good deal of royal imaginings. English writer Laurie Lee spent most of his decidedly poor village childhood convinced he was "something special, a young king perhaps placed secretly here in order to mix with the commoners. There is clearly a mystery about my birth, I feel so unique and majestic. One day, I know, the secret will be told." Today, a well-meaning therapist would soon cure him of these "delusions of grandeur." But that wouldn't be wise. Far better to define them as *realities* of grandeur, as they are natural manifestations of what researchers now consider a vital human sense: the sense of purpose. All of us have more in common with British royalty than we realize. As Michael Mann, Dean of Windsor, told the Queen, "this feeling of being set aside for a particular task" is universal.

The first to claim it with authority was famed psychologist Viktor Frankl. Writing in *Man's Search for Meaning* he argued: "Everyone has his own specific vocation or mission in life to carry out a concrete assignment which demands fulfillment. Therein he cannot be replaced, nor can his life be repeated. Thus, everyone's task is as unique as is his specific opportunity to implement it." Frankl knew what he was talking about. Survivor of a Nazi concentration camp, he witnessed the power of purpose firsthand, observing that the more his fellow prisoners realized and hung on to their unique purpose in life, the longer they were able to endure the hardships of the camp. Purpose wasn't just a rosy boost to self-esteem, it was crucial for survival. Since then, researchers have uncovered heaps of supporting evidence. Having a strong sense of purpose in life—a "devoir," as the Queen Mother would say—has been shown to increase your longevity, reduce your chances of a heart attack, boost your immune system and dramatically lessen your risk of developing Alzheimer's. And you hardly need a throne to cash in on the benefits. Purpose is so potent, the slightest increase can have stunning implications on mind and body. In a now classic experiment, when researchers gave elderly nursing home patients the simple duty of caring for a small houseplant in their room, which they were charged to nurture and watch grow, the patients' physical health and psychological well-being surged substantially. Remarkably, the patients were taking better care of *themselves* because they had some purpose, outside of themselves, to take care of.

This virtuous cycle has been evident in the Queen's life since the very beginning. On the sudden death of her father, the King, when her life changed forever, a strong sense of duty snapped into place, preventing Elizabeth from physically and emotionally collapsing. She spent what amounted to only a brief moment in private bewilderment, then was back at her desk drafting important documents within hours. "A slight flush on her face the only sign" that her world had just turned upside down, observed Martin Charteris. Princesses Margaret, on the other hand, heard the news and fell to pieces, took to her bed and required sedatives to calm her down. It goes without saying that Margaret, at the time, had very few royal duties to occupy her. The different responses are typical of what purpose—or a lack of it—can do for our inner stability. As Steve Taylor, senior lecturer in psychology at Leeds Beckett University in the UK, explains, "When you're 'in purpose'—that is, engaged with and working toward your purpose—life becomes easier, less complicated and stressful. You become more mono-focused, like an arrow flying toward its target, and your mind feels somehow taut and strong, with less space for negativity to seep in."

This was plainly evident in Elizabeth's personal transformation after she embraced her calling and assumed the throne. Previously shy and riddled with doubts about her youth and inexperience, Elizabeth the Queen "no longer [felt] anxious or worried," she told a friend. "I don't know what it is—but I have lost all my timidity somehow in becoming the Sovereign."

Anxiety and stress relief, to be sure, is one of the biggest links between purpose and better health. Challenges and complex decisions in life are far less daunting, distracting and blood-pressure soaring when you are guided by a clear purpose. Exactly how well this has benefited the Queen is pretty obvious when you consider how few sick days she has taken throughout her reign. "He who has a *why* to live for can bear with almost any *how*," as Nietzsche famously put it.

*

Prince Philip found this out the hard way. Beginning royal life with energetic purpose, enjoying a fulfilling and quickly advancing career in the Royal Navy, the King's untimely death drastically rerouted those plans. Putting his naval life on permanent hold, he became the Queen's consort, a vacuously vague position Philip once described as making him feel more like "a bloody amoeba" than a man. Without a definable role (or one he regarded as terribly important), Philip became decidedly mopey, quick-tempered and eventually seriously unwell. In his first year as consort, he came down with a severe case of jaundice—a condition often linked with stress and depression—and spent three agonizing weeks in a dark room trying to recover. But with few professional responsibilities to jump out of bed for, his recovery was predictably slow.*

Princess Margaret, as previously hinted, was another victim of the purposeless life. Aside from looking glamorous at royal events, Margaret had so few real obligations in life, her biographer Craig Brown notes that she frequently succumbed to cleaning her seashell collection out of pure boredom. One can't help but feel that caring for one of those nursing home houseplants would have been a marked improvement. "She has no direction, no overriding interest," observed the diarist Roy Strong, after a revealing evening spent with the princess in 1975. "All she likes now is *la jeunesse doré* and Young Men." Margaret clearly sensed this was wrong, but instead of addressing the problem, she chose to

---

* Viktor Frankl believed that a lack of purpose lay at the root of many forms of depression and emotional illnesses. As philanthropy expert Jenny Santi explains, "depression can result when the chasm between what a person is and what he ought to be becomes so vast . . . that something is seriously wrong and needs working through and changing." In other words, depression may be your biological signal that there is a real imbalance between the life you're living and your true purpose.

take it out on others, frequently lashing out in bitter resentment at her sister's stronger sense of direction. In one of her more famous attacks, Margaret interrupted a private meeting between the Queen and Prime Minister Harold Macmillan, barging into the room with the spiteful accusation "No one would talk to you if you weren't the Queen," before barging out again. For those who watched Margaret age into an ill and temperamental older woman, the price she paid for lacking a unique purpose was pitifully clear. Considering the depth of her untapped talents and potential, her obituary in the *Independent* could only lament that "the absence of a role was her tragedy." The real tragedy was that this was exactly what Margaret feared most. "I have always had a dread of becoming a passenger in life," she said. No one better understood the enormous risk of leaving one's purpose up to chance.

It might seem like Elizabeth (the lucky sister) received her well-defined purpose on a silver platter when her father died, but she had been proactively deciding what her "devoir" would be well before then. In 1947 at the age of 21, she did what many psychologists now advise: she created a personal purpose statement. "It is very simple," Elizabeth said in her first broadcast to the Commonwealth. "I declare before you all that my whole life, whether it be long or short, shall be devoted to your service and the service of our great imperial family to which we all belong." Short and sweet, but she has found daily clarity within its guidelines ever since. So important is this simple phrase to the Queen, it has been echoed on her Silver (1977), Golden (2002), and Diamond (2012) Jubilees—as much in reminder to herself as to her people. It is now her personal manifesto.

You might want to avoid the regal presumption of actually broadcasting it over the airwaves, but creating your own purpose statement can be incredibly helpful in figuring out how your special talents and interests come together to make you irreplaceably "unique and alone in the universe," as Viktor Frankl would say. Elizabeth might be lucky to have a purpose perfectly aligned with her actual job, but a true life purpose often has little to do with the means by which you earn your material salary. And it can justifiably take years to figure out.* Take it

---

* See *Life on Purpose* by Victor J. Strecher for some starting comparisons, including: "To live

from Prince Charles, somebody who's had to totally rethink his unique role as the longest-waiting heir apparent in British history. "I didn't suddenly wake up in my pram one day and say, 'Yippee,'" he said. "It just dawns on you . . . and slowly you get the idea that you have a certain duty and responsibility."

But a brief word on those duties and responsibilities (and Charles should probably pay attention to this): Research has shown that all purposes aren't created equal. For their fulfilling and life-lengthening powers to work, you'll need to avoid these common pitfalls. First, your purpose cannot be based on the pursuit of pleasure. It can *bring* pleasure, certainly, but pleasure cannot be its prime objective. Our brains are very good at differentiating between a noble purpose and one based on hedonistic self-gratification. And nature makes it pretty obvious which one it prefers. People who are driven by physical pleasures are more likely to have higher markers of inflammation, decreased immune responses and greater risk of depression than people driven by more selfless aims. Every pleasure-seeking monarch in history can confirm this. To rule just because you want all the land, all the food, all the gold or all the wives you could ever wish for always ends bad or sad . . . or fatally bloated. On the flip side, people can experience tremendous hardships and challenges and be psychologically protected if they are driven by higher ideals. Psychiatrist Anthony Clare believes this explains why so many Britons who lived through the struggles of World War II recall it as the best and healthiest years of their lives. "There was a shared philosophy, a common purpose," he says. "The basic fighting man felt he was doing something worthwhile. . . . And those engaged in the war were testing themselves. That seems to be rather important. Happy people are rarely sitting around. They are usually involved in some ongoing interchange of life." Which brings us to the second point: your purpose has to be bigger than yourself.

---

fully, experiencing each moment, aware, alert, and attentive" (Madeleine L'Engle, children's author); "To keep trying to understand a little more deeply the universe we are all in, to try to take one more step on this unending quest. And to have fun along the way" (Ronald Graham, mathematician); "To relieve suffering and to exercise compassion" (Harry Blackmun, US Supreme Court Justice); "To put a ding in the universe" (Steve Jobs).

"This is the true joy in life," wrote George Bernard Shaw, "the being used for a purpose recognized by yourself as a mighty one." If you don't think your purpose is mighty enough, that it matters to someone other than yourself, it won't be what gets you out of bed in the morning. Though the Queen would be the first to point out that "mighty" is a relative term here. "Remember that good spreads outward and every little does help. Mighty things from small beginnings grow," said Elizabeth in a 1976 broadcast, using one of her favorite metaphors, that of dropping pebbles into a pond. "A big stone can cause waves, but even the smallest pebble changes the whole pattern of the water. Our daily actions are like those ripples, each one makes a difference, even the smallest . . . And the combined effect can be enormous."

Every worthy purpose, duty, calling, destiny or "devoir" begins there, with the carefully considered question: what will be my own ripples, and will they still benefit others long after I am gone? Continuity is key.* Everyone you have ever deeply admired has lived by this maxim. Just imagine if J. R. R. Tolkien or Mother Teresa or Benjamin Franklin went in for early retirement. To "resign" from the legacy you alone can fulfill is to let far more than yourself down. In Elizabeth's case, this includes an entire kingdom which, let's be honest, still isn't quite ready for the reign of King Charles III. *Vive le devoir!*

---

* Unsurprisingly, "continuity" is the single most repeated word when the Queen's legacy is described by politicians, archbishops, senior civil servants and her own family, according to Andrew Marr.

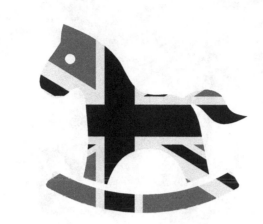

Play Like a Queen

I'm afraid Her Majesty is getting to be
what is known as a handful.

—ALAN BENNETT, *THE UNCOMMON READER*

R oyal teenagers will be teenagers. In the summer of 1998, Prince William and Harry thought it would be fun to spend the day at Grywne-Fawr dam in Wales and—will you look at that wicked incline!—strap themselves into harnesses and abseil down the 160-foot dam wall. Probably having the time of their lives, the princes were spotted by a concerned passerby who promptly showed her genuine distress by snapping a photo of Harry suspended over the man-made cliff and selling the image to the highest media bidder. Because as everyone knows, if the media loathes and abominates one thing, it's an accident waiting to happen. Noticing Harry wasn't wearing the proper safety gear, cries of "madness" and "foolhardy" filled the headlines. "It's not every day that you see the future king and his brother going over the edge of a sheer drop," reported the *News of the World*. It seemed the Windsors had recklessly parted company with their brain cells. Charles was furious, and the nanny in charge came dangerously close to losing her job.* Even the Royal Society for the Prevention of Accidents put in their parental two cents. Their grandmother the Queen, however, remained oddly quiet, apart from a dry statement from Buckingham Palace that amounted to *yes, yes, safety first and we'll try a bit harder next time.* It was obvious the Queen's heart wasn't in it. Harry and William might have been a tad overenthusiastic, but there was little chance Elizabeth would criticize the essence of what has been so crucial in her own life: play.

---

* Fondly known as "Tiggy" to the princes (after the Beatrix Potter character, Mrs. Tiggy-winkle), Alexandra Legge-Bourke had an impressive knack for getting into comical scrapes. That same year, a paparazzi shot emerged of her driving a royal vehicle around the Balmoral estate, a cigarette dangling in her mouth, while Prince Harry, age fourteen, leaned out of the window shooting rabbits. Evidently Tiggy was putting her own unique spin on Beatrix Potter's credo: "If I have done anything—even a little—to help small children on the road to enjoy and appreciate honest simple pleasures . . . I have done a bit of good."

This side of Her Majesty can seriously stump the general public. A Queen at work rifling through her red boxes, dutifully meeting the masses and solemnly handing out honors and awards is what we're used to. It would hardly be surprising to hear that she bestows knighthoods in her sleep. But that's not the full portrait. As her family, friends and anyone who has witnessed the mischievous sparkle in her eye can attest, Elizabeth can just as accurately be defined as a Queen at play. Showing a rare spark of mindful immaturity, Elizabeth has preserved and nurtured a habit most of us have lost to childhood. Where play is concerned, the Queen has essentially never grown up. From four to ninety-four, play has been the natural outlet for her wider passions, her means of exercise, her mental rejuvenation and her preferred mode of physical rest. And as we'll soon see, she wouldn't be the focused, hardworking and long-lived Queen without it. To quote her first private secretary, Tommy Lascelles, Elizabeth has "a healthy sense of fun" in the truest sense of the expression.

You might even say that "play" itself has kept the monarchy flourishing into the twenty-first century—something which endlessly confounds its critics. Whenever there's a big royal celebration, jubilee or wedding, media pundits predict certain doom for the Crown. Once the public sees how much this frivolity is going to cost, they say, people will rant and rebel and insist the expensive merrymaking stops. They are *always* proven wrong. The universal instinct for play is too strong. In fact, rather than grabbing for their pitchforks in mass rebellion, the public wildly appreciate these royal reminders to take time off work, to let loose over a coronation cup of punch and wave their mini Union Jacks with all the shameless fervor of a six-year-old. Winston Churchill understood the impulse well. It's how he justified the cost of Elizabeth and Philip's wedding in 1947, smack in the middle of a period of severe economic austerity in Britain after World War II. More frugality, more grinding work, was the last thing people needed, he thought, insisting that a frivolous "flash of colour on the hard road we have to travel" would do everyone far more good in the long run. He was, and continues to be, absolutely right.

HER MAJESTY'S
PLEASURE

OR RULE #9—ONE MUSTN'T
STOP HORSING AROUND

It made him remember his first childhood vividly,
the happy times swimming in moats or flying with Archimedes,
and he realised that he had lost something since those days.
It was something which he thought of now as the faculty of wonder.
—T. H. WHITE, *THE ONCE AND FUTURE KING*

E lizabeth came dangerously close to being a very unplayful
Queen. A naturally reserved child with an innate awareness of
life's duties far beyond her years, her displays of restraint could
reach nun-like proportions, especially in the playroom. She had what
amounted to an existential play crisis at age nine. It was the winter
of 1936 and the country was mourning the death of King George V.
Considered too young to attend "Grandpa England's" funeral, Elizabeth
spent the intervening hours with Margaret in the nursery, playing with
her beloved toy horses. It was a pastime Elizabeth deeply enjoyed, but
she couldn't help but wonder, was this what a dutiful princess should be
doing? Turning to her governess with a marked tone of anxiety, Elizabeth
blurted out, "Oh, Crawfie . . . ought we to play?" Prepared to sacrifice

pleasure on the altar of royal propriety, Elizabeth (nine going on ninety) waited for the reply that could have been the nail in her serious coffin. Fate, however, was mercifully kind. Crawfie reassured Elizabeth that play was not only appropriate at the moment, her grandfather would never have wanted her to stop. "The last thing anyone you loved would wish you to do was to sit round and be miserable," said Crawfie. From that moment something seemed to click. Elizabeth never questioned the need for play in her life again.

There was the additional boon, of course, of having parents who prioritized play and a spirited sister in Princess Margaret—acting as self-appointed court jester—who laughed Elizabeth out of her natural reserve. Despite a four-year age difference, little was made of the gap, and they were each other's closest playmates. Elizabeth's own years of childhood play would be greatly extended as she waited for Margaret to catch up. It was an unquestionably idyllic time. They gamboled through the English and Scottish countryside playing games like "catching the days" (catching autumn leaves as they fell from trees) and joined their parents in the evening for wild romps with playing cards that left everyone blissfully panting for breath. Elizabeth was still pretending and putting on pantomime shows with Margaret well into her teenage years. At seventeen and already technically dating Prince Philip, she looked years younger cavorting on stage with her sister in the Windsor Castle production of *Aladdin*, featuring achingly silly dialogue and (why wasn't I there to see this?) a snappy tap dance number from the future Queen.

Yet there's no evidence that Elizabeth suffered any teenage angst or embarrassment for doing so. Play seemed perfectly natural. In fact, she's a classic case of the normalcy of childhood play overlapping into young adulthood. What's *abnormal* is losing it—sadly something the majority of us will experience sometime in early adolescence. The pressure of peer groups is frightfully effective at squelching our innate childhood sense of play. Faced with new social constructs that play is somehow uncool, immature or unproductive, few children are able to retain their unique relationship with play into their teenage years—a setback most adults never recover from. Elizabeth wasn't among them. Remarkably, her formative years were virtually absent of peer pressure. In what has to be conceded as producing unquestionably healthy results, the King and Queen sheltered her from anyone or anything that might pressure her to conform to ideas contrary to her inner self. So Elizabeth blithely kept on playing. And she really never stopped.

Even in her nineties the Queen can be "positively girlish . . . [and] childlike," says body language expert Judi James, one of many eyewitnesses to Elizabeth's playful spirit. Like the time she sailed from Bermuda to the US on the rocky yacht *Britannia*. Rough seas had left most of the royal party, including navy man Prince Philip, feeling nauseously "grey and grim," reported Susan Crosland, wife of the foreign secretary. The Queen, however, was relishing every minute of it. Her long chiffon scarf flying in the wind, she grabbed hold of a sliding door and, as a large swell lifted the ship, let out a long "Wheeeeee!" while sliding across the floor as the door slammed shut. Ronald and Nancy Reagan also saw Elizabeth's inner child unleashed. On a 1983 visit to their ranch in California, located high atop the Santa Ynez Mountain range, record rainfall had all but washed out the seven-mile road up to the ranch. But instead of calling off the visit, the Queen decided to abandon her limousine at the base of the mountain, squeeze into a tiny Jeep and brave the dangerous ascent. Arriving wet and noticeably crinkled, the Reagans apologized profusely for the inconvenience. "Don't be silly!" replied Elizabeth. "This is an adventure!"

On the job, the Queen can turn her normally plodding work with politicians into a form of play. In a private game some have called "catching out the minister," the Queen will prepare extra carefully for her weekly audience with the prime minister to see if she can surprise him with an overlooked (though important) piece of government news. She famously played Winston Churchill in this way, who once failed to familiarize himself with an important cable from the British ambassador in Iraq. "What did you think about that most interesting telegram from Baghdad?" asked the Queen. Churchill admitted his ignorance and returned to his office thoroughly displeased with his secretaries, but with a newfound respect for the young Queen. It wouldn't be the last time her childlike sense of play, ironically, increased her standing as a

serious, responsible adult. All thanks to the wonders of—if I may brave
a little-known technical term—*neoteny*.

＊

From the Greek for "stretch" or "extend," neoteny is any characteristic
of childhood that stretches into adult life. Many species retain juvenile
features after maturity (consider the pygmy chimpanzee), but humans
have the rare capacity to embrace neoteny on purpose, primarily through
play. Eighty-some-year-old play expert Dr. Stuart Brown believes it to be
one of our most beneficial and untapped biological faculties. Studying
play behaviors in nature, he noticed that animals that retain a sense of
play remain, in a cerebral sense, "forever young"—their brains are more
adaptive to new challenges than creatures that abandon play in adulthood. Domesticated wolves (i.e., dogs), explicitly bred to remain playful
throughout their lives, are the classic example. Whereas a wild wolf will
stop playing early in life, becoming locked in an increasingly narrow
set of compulsive behaviors, old dogs can still learn new tricks. They
are essentially wolf puppies in a permanent holding pattern, retaining a
sense of curiosity about the world and a sustained ability to learn new
behaviors, far and above what an adult wolf could ever manage. Play
appears to suspend the brain in its earliest, most plastic stage of development. Which explains why crossover studies in humans are now finding
strong links between adult play and the prevention of neurological
diseases, like dementia and Alzheimer's.

The Queen Mother had an iconic handle on this. Nicknamed
"Merry Mischief" as a child, she never abandoned her playful (or,
what she called, "naughty") spirit and had a serious suspicion it is
what got her, still smiling, to her 101st birthday. "I love life. That's the
secret," she said, when pressed to explain her extraordinary longevity.
"It is the exhilaration of others that keeps me going. Sometimes I feel
drained, you do at my age, but excitement is good for me." Spending
two years working as the Queen Mother's equerry in the mid-nineties,
Major Colin Burgess left the position crammed full of memories of
her "naughty" escapades. Though pushing ninety-five at the time, she
still wanted to ride a motorbike in her back garden or zoom incognito
through the streets of London in a friend's sports car. Prince William

and Harry reportedly taught her how to play video games, and she once (presumably inspired by Annie Oakley) playfully considered bringing a firearm to her outdoor luncheons, in order to pop off the troublesome squirrels between courses. Through it all the Queen Mother expressed, what Stuart Browns calls, her personal "play history"—connecting her to the dimpled Merry Mischief of her past and keeping her mind agile to the very end. She never lost her "utterly irresistible mischievousness of spirit," said her favorite grandchild, Prince Charles—nor, as others have noted, her wicked skills for cheating at card games.*

Examining her daughter's life, we find the same unbroken play continuum. As a girl, if Elizabeth wasn't spending hours grooming and saddling her toy horses, she was pretending to be one. "We cavorted endlessly at horses," said her cousin Margaret Rhodes, recalling life in the royal nursery. "We galloped round and round. We were horses of every kind: carthorses, racehorses and circus horses. We spent a lot of time as circus horses and it was obligatory to neigh." In a scene straight out of *National Velvet*, Crawfie (newly appointed as governess) first met Elizabeth bouncing about in bed, a mop-topped girl around seven years old, "busy driving her team" of imaginary horses strapped to the bedposts by the cords of her dressing gown. Asked if this was a nightly habit, Elizabeth replied with all seriousness, "I mostly go once or twice round the park before I go to sleep, you know. It exercises my horses." Crawfie was soon prancing about herself, harnessed as a grocer's carthorse, while Elizabeth delivered imaginary goods around the nursery.

Your childhood was likely one large sandbox of similar consuming passions—either for Barbies, Legos, dinosaurs or toy cars—but few have made the play transition into adulthood so seamlessly as Elizabeth. Simply exchanging the imaginary for the real, the Queen still plays with horses on a daily basis, either through visiting her stables yards,

---

* A play history which was instilled and nurtured by her own mother, Lady Strathmore. Widely read and interested in childhood development, Lady Strathmore admired the teachings of Friedrich Froebel, the nineteenth-century German educator and creator of kindergartens, who believed unfettered play was integral to children's mental growth. Quite advanced for a time when children were, more often, expected to be seen and not heard.

expanding her encyclopedic knowledge of breeding and bloodlines, cheering her thoroughbreds at the racecourse or riding her Fell ponies around the Windsor estate (shorter and easier for her to mount now in older age). Elizabeth might not be as equinely obsessed as her daughter, Princess Anne, whose interests, Prince Philip famously remarked, extend only to what flatulates and eats hay, but the Queen will light up more over a conversation about horses than any discussion about the Commonwealth. It's "the one subject she can get deeply immersed in," said her former stud manager Michael Oswald, "that is completely divorced from her everyday work."

Horses are the Queen's "heart play," to use a charming term coined by motivational speaker and play convert Barbara Brannen, who believes that what was magical, engrossing and inspiring to us as children is very likely still beckoning us as adults. Not simply what amuses or distracts you, "heart play" is what you gravitated to naturally as a child, a unique expression of play and pleasure so deeply embedded in one's personality, Brannen is convinced that a healthy adult life (to say nothing of a creative or happy one) is impossible without retaining some form of it. For Brannen, it was reconnecting with her childhood joy in the great outdoors, but it can, she points out, be practically anything that once fired your imagination and still makes "your heart sing and fly free," creating "an ecstasy that may not be apparent to anyone but you." If this sounds a bit too irresponsibly millennial / Silicon Valley / adult playground / hipster to you, it's worth remembering that the enormously productive psychiatrist Carl Jung felt compelled to start playing with building blocks again at the age of 38, tapping into a childhood pastime that reignited his mental energy and enthusiasm for work, a decision Jung later described as "a turning point in my fate." More recently, influential psychologist Mihaly Csikszentmihalyi discovered that playful activities are one of the easiest ways to trigger the optimal mental condition known as "flow"—a focused state of pleasure with enormous capabilities to trigger creativity and greater well-being. Anthropologists now speak of the brain-boosting power of "deep play," clearly distancing themselves from the playground version. But it's all just *play* in the end. And as the title of Stuart Brown's TED Talk makes clear, "Play is more than just fun."*

*

First, whether it takes the form of a hobby or a passion, the intrinsic joy of play makes it an inexhaustible source of positivity, countering the grimmer realities of adult life. Elizabeth's former racing manager, Lord Carnarvon, believed that talking about horses almost every day to the Queen brought tremendous balance to her psyche. "Her responsibilities as monarch," he explained, mean that "most of the news she gets is bad. That someone has died or some accident has happened or something else unpleasant." In the Queen's stables, however, there's almost always something to take pride or pleasure in. "When the horses run well, the right sexed foal has been born, it's a bit of an uplift to her," said Carnarvon. "One feels one is giving her a bit of good news for once." Yet even if the Queen's horse doesn't win a prized race—and she has endured many defeats on the turf—the long-term pleasure in mastering a passion overrides any temporary disappointments. Play is the only human endeavor where we can repeatedly fail and still have fun in the process. This was one of the persistent warning signs in Princess Diana's adult life. She had no discernable hobbies and no diverting pastimes outside her risky toying and teasing of the British press, which occasionally turned remorselessly against her. "She was an empty vessel, a pretty empty vessel, but empty nonetheless," admitted her longtime confidant Michael Colborne. With no way of playfully balancing life's negativity and increasingly incapable of spending any time alone, solitude for Diana meant only boredom or crushing loneliness. Bearing out one of the harsher realities of play deprivation: "the opposite of play is not work, it's depression," says Stuart Brown.

---

* Elizabeth's uncle David—briefly King Edward VIII—never quite understood the distinction. Though he believed he was perpetually boyish, like many adults he confused real *play* with the typical triad of adult amusements: partying, drinking and sex (usually to excess), things which have nothing at all to do with one's inner "heart play." As every child knows, candy is nice, but it's not play.

Second, play is preparatory. In T. H. White's Arthurian classic *The Once and Future King*, the wizard Merlin uses play as the medium through which young Arthur learns the art of kingship. For good reason. Play is the easiest way to mentally prepare for future challenges. One of the true wonders of "heart play" is how well it predicts what personalized skills your adult self will need, be it resilience, bravery, determination or diplomacy. The latter certainly applied in Queen Victoria's case. Though her childhood was far removed from the court life she would one day inhabit, Victoria was drawn to a specific form of play that provided daily practice for her later role as Queen and Empress. What toy horses were to Elizabeth, dolls were to Victoria. She had more than a hundred of them, through which, we are told, "she rehearsed court receptions, presentations, and held mimic drawing-room levees"—all gradually preparing her, one day, for the real thing on an epically imperial scale. People who criticize the current Queen's horsing pursuits as a waste of time usually run into the same argument. Especially after the extreme calmness she showed in 1982, when an emotionally deranged intruder broke into her bedroom and decided to have a suicidal chat with her alone (whilst holding a broken and bloodied shard of glass). Suddenly the Queen's lifelong play habit seemed entirely justified. All those years calming spooked and frightened horses had been practice well spent. "Riding taught [her] to be cool in a crisis," one journalist deduced.*

Play is so good at sharpening our wits, we become more creative when we enter a childlike state of play, as one study out of North Dakota State University revealed. When two groups of college students were given the same creative task to complete, one group significantly outperformed the other. Yet the only difference between the groups was imaginative play. Whereas the first group was simply told to begin the

---

* Interestingly, this is the whole premise behind horse or "equine" therapy, a form of therapeutic play which has helped countless troubled teens and emotionally wounded veterans regain a sense of inner equilibrium. Since horses have a skittish sixth sense for erratic behavior, people engaged in equine therapy are forced to practice a level of mental calm most have never fully tapped into before, a process that can be deeply healing. After the embarrassment of her "Fake Sheikh" scandal in 2010, Sarah Ferguson turned to equine therapy to stop her emotional world from reeling.

task, the higher-scoring group was first instructed to imagine they were playful seven-year-olds with lots of free time on their hands. Play made all the difference. This is why daily recess is of such extreme cognitive value for children, despite recently being squeezed out of school curriculums in favor of "higher" academic pursuits. Yet when children are given ample time and space for unstructured, nonproductive play, studies have found that they become smarter, more attentive students in the classroom. Such wisdom clearly runs deep in the Windsor consciousness. The first charity William and Harry financially supported was the Queen Elizabeth II Fields Challenge, which seeks to protect Britain's green spaces and playing fields from being concreted over by developers. It was also one of the first charitable causes Philip took on in 1949.

Finally, play is healing. Though she might have questioned the impulse at the time, the upsetting death of her grandfather naturally prompted Elizabeth to play, lovingly grooming her toy horses. "You couldn't feel properly sad with a brush in one hand and the other on a horse's neck," says biographer Elizabeth Longford. The reflex is almost universal. Children turn to play after traumatic events with the same reactionary speed that many adults turn to therapists. But it has little to do with coping through distraction. For children especially, play provides a rare sense of feeling in control. Whereas the wider world can be a terrifying hodgepodge of unpredictable and seemingly random events, play is the safe (and oftentimes only) place where they fully understand the rules. Every playground in the world bears this out. What may seem like absolute anarchy to an outsider is actually a microcosm of well-defined boundaries and unspoken laws, usually confirmed by one child screaming "that's not fair!" More sensitive children will naturally gravitate to pretend play for this reason. They can blissfully make up the rules of their own world as they go along. And it doesn't appear we ever outgrow the need for it. Play, through an adult hobby or passion, enables us to slip into a world where the rules are refreshingly clear-cut or entirely of our own making. Mihaly Csikszentmihalyi calls it the "Paradox of Control." Quite distinct from ordinary life, "where any number of bad things can happen," says Csikszentmihalyi, play is a minimal risk zone. If you're constructing a tower of building blocks, the worst that can happen is to see it tumble down. In a world no less crazy and unpredictable for adults, this sense of control can be massively therapeutic. It's one of the rare areas of life where Prince Charles, surprisingly, has followed in his mother's footsteps. Speaking of his lifelong love for painting with watercolors and galloping about on the polo field, Charles describes play as transporting him "into another dimension which, quite literally, refreshes parts of the soul which other activities can't reach." It's "one of the best ways I know," he said, "of forgetting the pressures and complications of life."

If you want an even better reason to resurrect your inner child and start horsing around again, consider the parting wisdom of Queen Mary. Always driven by a relentless sense of duty (and more tightly laced than the ossified woman at the sideshow), she had but one poignant regret as her exhaustively industrious life drew to a close. Confiding to her daughter-in-law, she unbuttoned one of her innermost secrets: "Do you know there is one thing I never did and wish I had done: climbed over a fence!"

FIT TO RULE

OR RULE #10—I HEREBY BANISH
MAD EXERCISE

Horses sweat, gentlemen perspire,
but ladies only gently glow.
—Victorian saying

The room was hot and crowded. Both women had been on their feet for hours. Packed with 1,000 guests tussling for a chance to meet the prime minister and monarch, the annual diplomatic reception at Buckingham Palace can be a grueling event at the best of times. But this year a pronounced whiff of competition hung in the air. Acting as Britain's first "elected" queen (somewhat overcompensating for her social inferiority complex), Margaret Thatcher was attempting to impress the crowd with the steely persona that would one day earn her the title of "Iron Lady." But as the real Queen sailed serenely through the sea of ambassadors, cabinet ministers and officials of church and state, Thatcher was finding it hard to keep up. The room was stifling, her feet ached, her head was woozy with small talk and after one handshake too many, she all but fainted onto a nearby chair. Apparently her iron needed time to harden. The following year, she would get another try. But again, Thatcher couldn't quite make it to the party finish line. For the second year running, and with hundreds of diplomats still waiting in the wings, she collapsed in a pale, exhausted heap. Glancing across the room, the Queen simply noted, "Oh look!

She's keeled over again," before resuming her steady course around the assembled guests. Elizabeth moved through the crowd "like a liner," noted an impressed onlooker that evening. It was all-too obvious who the real Iron Lady was.

Thatcher wasn't the first to match muscle against Her Majesty and lose, nor would she be the last. Perhaps more misjudged than any of the Queen's personal attributes is that under her deceptively petite figure is a fireball of stamina and inexhaustible energy. "I'm as strong as a horse," Elizabeth likes to say to those who suggest she might need a rest. Long ago her grandmother Queen Mary warned her that the job would entail endless hours on her feet, and she has risen to the physical challenge.* Elizabeth's endurance is "striking," says biographer Sally Bedell Smith, who recounts the time the Queen was touring Canada when, after a long day of tightly packed events, the tour organizer suddenly realized he had not given the Queen one moment's break, not even to use the loo. "You need not worry," said her private secretary. "Her Majesty is trained for eight hours." The Queen likewise never sits at Palace events, unless it's a dinner, and always stands during her Privy Council meetings. Small wonder then, in a rare slip of personal detail, one of her private secretaries acknowledged that among the Queen's "great assets" is her "very good legs . . . she can stand for a long time." Those who wish to accompany the Queen have to keep pace. A little-known require-ment of becoming a lady-in-waiting to Her Majesty is the ability to stand for hours without tiring, oftentimes going without food or drink. Trained bodyguards have been known to tire in the wake of her limitless vigor. During a state visit to the Bush White House in the early 1990s, the president congratulated the Queen on doing something few people far younger had achieved. Her bracing walking speed had "left even the Secret Service panting," he joked. To use a well-worn phrase often applied to the Kings and Queens of England, but never so well justified, Elizabeth II is quite literally *fit to rule*.

---

* "My grandmother warned me I would have to stand for hours"—an injunction that likely occurred after Elizabeth, aged eleven, experienced what a full royal day could entail at her father's coronation in 1937. "When we sat down to tea it was nearly six o'clock!" she wrote. "When I got into bed my legs ached terribly!"

Though you'd be hard-pressed to find the word "workout" in any biography of the Queen. She has never lifted a dumbbell, hopped on an elliptical, tracked her heart rate or done anything resembling a squat, lunge, crunch, press or curl in a gym environment. The only real "weight training" Elizabeth has ever endured was done out of regal necessity. Insisting on wearing the traditional (and cumbersomely heavy) St. Edward's Crown for her coronation in 1953, Elizabeth rehearsed for weeks prior, marching around the Palace wearing the nearly five-pound jewel-encrusted crown, priming her neck muscles for the big event. Employees in the Palace kitchen liken it to carrying two bags of sugar on your head. It's an upper-body exercise that repeats every year at the State Opening of Parliament, when she usually dons an even heavier crown and power-strolls to her throne under the fifteen-pound velvet Robe of State. But the Queen isn't keen on repeating the exertion more than necessary.*

Prince Philip has always been the bigger exercise aficionado of the two, though some might say *addict*. Neurotically weight conscious, Philip used to pile on two or three sweaters and go for intense runs around the royal grounds whenever he thought an unwelcome pound had materialized on his body. A restless "dynamo" to his friends, Philip "crackled with energy," but often didn't know when to stop. Sprinting from one intense sport or workout to the next, he'd return to the Queen's rooms so exhausted, he'd be forced to lie down. "I think Prince Philip is mad," said Elizabeth to a member of staff, watching her husband dart out of the door in yet another attempt to "work up a sweat." For the Queen, it frankly bordered on the insane.

She sees nothing pleasant in being painfully "puffed," as she calls it, immensely preferring a calm walk instead. The Queen "is a great believer in sensible exercise," says biographer Ingrid Seward, noting that apart from gentle gallops on her horses and a few occasional country sports, walking has been the one constant source of physical activity in

---

* In 2019 Elizabeth finally decided to swap out the seven-pound Imperial State Crown for the lighter George IV Diadem at the Opening of Parliament. Looking down to read the speech had become ergonomically perilous, explained the Queen, "because if you did, your neck would break; it would fall off."

her life. When at Buckingham Palace, every afternoon around two thirty she'll go for a long walk around the gardens with her corgis. Out in the country, at Balmoral or Sandringham, she'll ramble a bit longer through moorlands and woods. But nothing designates these times as particularly exercisey in nature. There are no fancy sneakers or fast-swishing arm movements to speak of. Elizabeth simply walks naturally, with an "intentionally measured and deliberate pace," to quote her longtime dress designer Norman Hartnell. She will, perhaps, wear wellies and carry a walking stick if feeling particularly adventurous. But little else is involved in exercising like a Queen. Meanwhile, the Buckingham Palace gym is "rarely used except by a handful of sweating footmen," says journalist Tina Brown.

*

It might be easier to accept if Elizabeth admitted to concealing a high-intensity cardio trainer in the Palace attic. Prince Philip's longevity, after all, is so much easier to explain because of his more traditional (read rigorous) approach to fitness. But despite being almost universally accepted as fact, research has never supported the *sweat more, strain more, live long* formula. On the contrary, studies of lifestyle patterns in blue zones around the world (where life-spans are highest), show a surprising reversal of typical gym-like behaviors. Whereas the "healthiest" souls in America pound their joints, muscles, tendons and hearts in feverish spurts a few times a week, people in blue zones show a marked preference for more moderate activities. On the Italian island of Sardinia, longevity researcher Dan Buettner noticed that people most likely to reach their one-hundredth birthday were those who simply walked and moved more every day, not necessarily more strenuously. Shepherds tending their flocks, slowly meandering up and down the Sardinian hillsides on foot, had the highest chance of becoming centenarians, more so than farmers in the same population (people more likely to damage and inflame their joints through more strenuous labor). The discovery led Buettner to abandon the exercise mania of modern gyms in favor of more "regular, low-intensity physical effort" of the sort traditionally embraced in blue zone regions: "the type of exercise that the rest of us should be doing." Buettner insists, "You'll never see me doing CrossFit," for the same reason you won't see Her Majesty engaged in any form of "mad" exercise, however much Philip has enticed her with the pungent delights of sweating in one's sweater.*

Then again, Philip and Elizabeth come from very different exercise backgrounds. Philip was heavily influenced by his education at Gordonstoun, a spartan-like boarding school in northern Scotland founded on a robust physical fitness philosophy and the rather exhausting motto "More is in you." The school day began with a freezing cold shower at six thirty and a run through the damp grounds (wearing only shorts, even in the winter). There was more running, jumping and javelin throwing before lunch, marine sports or construction projects in the afternoon and, in summer, rounds of tennis before bed. The boys who complained about the "training" (Philip was never one of them) found little sympathy from their stern German headmaster, Kurt Hahn. It was all for their own good, Hahn believed: "I should think as little of asking them whether they want to train, as I should think of asking them whether they feel in the mood to brush their teeth."

Meanwhile, Elizabeth was brought up believing there was little difference between being playfully active and being physically fit—a mentality largely nurtured by her father, King George VI. Remembering his own boot camp–style upbringing (and the physical rigors of the Royal Naval College as a thirteen-year-old cadet, complete with cold baths and floggings), George VI wanted something different for his beloved daughters. Namely, fun. He hired Marion Crawford as the girls' governess based on little more than the fact that she "loved walking" and seemed spry and "young enough to enjoy playing games and running about" with the princesses. Forever hatching up new ways to expend their energy, Crawfie took Margaret and Elizabeth to public pools in London and soon got them involved in Girl Guides, with its weekly meetings emphasizing outdoor games and activities. They went on mile-long marches with their troop through the Windsor Grounds, stood

---

* The Queen perspires so little, in fact, her ability to remain looking perpetually cool is somewhat of a regal phenomenon. On a 2010 visit to Ground Zero in New York, while everyone else was dripping in 103-degree heat, Elizabeth looked serenely fresh. "She didn't have a bead of sweat on her," said a dazzled bystander. "I thought that is what it must be like to be royal."

to attention, gathered wood for camping trips and took part in limb-stretching calisthenics. The meetings were invigorating but "only mildly strenuous," says biographer Carolly Erickson, and it was difficult to tell where the play ended and the exercise began.

For the most part, this is the typical childhood experience (disregarding the anomaly of British boarding schools). We only start artificially dissecting play and exercise as adults. Consider Sarah Ferguson's self-advice as a spokesperson for Weight Watchers International in the late 1990s. Writing in the (I must admit) gloriously titled *Dieting with the Duchess*, Sarah pens what might just be the saddest statement in the history of health manuals. "Exercise is different from activity," she insists. "Activity reminds me of children playing: moving, jumping, running or just doing something that is fun and spirited. Exercise, on the other hand, can be a chore. But it is imperative for your well-being." In other words, activity is jolly good fun, but it isn't *real* exercise. But what's that old saying? Oh yes—Don't believe everything a Duchess tells you.

*

"Our movement intensity does not have to be 'vigorous' or make us sweat to 'count,'" says behavioral scientist Michelle Segar, someone on the front lines of debunking fitness myths at the University of Michigan. "An almost infinite variety of physical movement choices and intensities will work just as well, or better, than a strict regimen of intense workouts—especially when people have chosen activities they actually enjoy doing." The knowledge has been there for decades, admits Segar, pointing to a 1996 report from the US Surgeon General which drastically redefined the official recommendations for physical fitness—from something done intensely at a specific time to something that could be divided up throughout the day through low-intensity activities. "But getting people to believe it, even today," says Segar, "is an uphill battle."

It's easier to understand when you consider the biological wonders of NEAT (non-exercise activity thermogenesis)—a fancy word scientists at Mayo Clinic use to describe all the energy you burn when you're not strictly "working out," but you're not sitting down either. It's everyday things like climbing stairs, doing the dishes, gardening, walking, or just plain fidgeting. And the accumulated caloric burn can add up substantially. Simple increases in NEAT activities can be "profoundly more powerful than going to the gym three times a week," says Dr. James Levine, a leading researcher in the field. It's one of the main reasons why children (who aren't stuck inside playing video games) remain so enviously trim and why adults who naturally engage in more daily NEAT actions seem almost inoculated against developing obesity.*

The mystery of Elizabeth's enduring fitness becomes clearer with this in mind. Especially when you consider the accumulated energy involved in simply walking around her homes and office—to say nothing of her frequent public "walkabouts." Amazed at the scale of Windsor Castle, Sarah Ferguson (a.k.a., Deceptive Duchess) admits that traversing its corridors of endless rooms can be "a major bit of exercise." Ditto the immense floor plan of Buckingham Palace. Crawfie felt it was "all far too big" and famously said that living there was like permanently camping in a museum. No slowpoke herself, Crawfie estimated that whenever she and the princesses wanted to take a walk in the garden, it took them a good five minutes just to get outside of the nearly 700-room Palace. "People here need bicycles," Elizabeth observed, shortly after moving in. The realities of NEAT further explain why the Queen's main sources of fun throughout her life (horseback riding, deer stalking, grouse shooting) while still counting as exercise have rarely left her "puffed"—a simple detail that has arguably made all the difference in her lifelong physical health.

Because despite the widespread belief that intense workouts release a steady flow of pleasurable endorphins, research has shown that exercise and pleasure actually coexist at a much lower range of physical intensity. The cut-off point appears to be anything *above* the "ventilation

---

* In a seminal study out of Mayo Clinic, Dr. Levine had volunteers eat 1,000 additional daily calories for 56 days (the rough equivalent of eating two *extra* Big Macs every day) while wearing specialized belts that would track their slightest movements. The difference between those who moved regularly throughout the day and those who predominantly stayed seated was astonishing. "People who have the ability to switch on their NEAT movement do not gain fat with overfeeding; they stay slim," reported Levine. "People who stay seated when they overfeed, and don't switch on their NEAT movement, deposit all the extra calories into body fat."

threshold," the point at which holding a conversation becomes impossible without panting for breath. And according to exercise psychologists, this is when, for most people, "pleasure" and "exercise" part company. Since this is the *exact* threshold most gyms and cardio sessions are so keen on getting us to cross, it's little wonder that most people are naturally not amused by modern workouts, and engage in them sporadically at best.* A few stalwart souls push through, like Prince Philip and Princess Diana, but their exercising tends to take on the unhealthy hallmarks of a compulsive behavior. Diana was manic about her early morning visits to the gym and pounding out a high number of laps in the pool. Exercise had become "an obsession for her," according to her friend-turned-lover James Hewitt. And she often crawled out of the pool more cranky and standoffish than when she got in. The Queen, however, will usually return from a quiet walk with her corgis more refreshed and renewed by the activity, ready to take on the next monarchial crisis.

*

Play and exercise are undoubtedly the most natural partners. When a subway station in Sweden sought to motivate more passengers to take the stairs rather than the adjacent escalator, they didn't put up motivational fitness signs but cleverly turned the process into a game. Transforming the staircase into a giant electric keyboard, researchers watched in amazement as 66 percent more people skipped the escalator to hop up and down the musical stairs. "Fun is the easiest way to change people's behavior for the better," said a spokesperson for the idea. Dog owners, for instance, consistently get more exercise than people who go to the gym simply because they find dog walking more enjoyable. That's the paradox of physical fitness. Long-term goals like "weight loss" a "better body" or "longevity," while entirely sensible, can't compete with the immediate rewards of active play. Exercise, like any life activity, is most easily sustained, says Michelle Segar, "when we view it as a gift, something that is fun or personally meaningful."

Take it from the Queen. The only physical activities Elizabeth has

---

* On average, people drop out of strict exercise programs after six months, and an estimated 67 percent of gym memberships go unused.

stuck with for decades are the ones that have brought her emotional pleasure. She relies on her daily walks and horseback rides, not because they have kept her muscles strengthened over the years (which they certainly have) but because they are her principal "alone" time, says biographer Christopher Andersen, when her mind gets a moment's rest from the demands of an ever-tightening Crown.* The health benefits are simply an added bonus. Though the resulting stamina of a woman who has uniquely "exercised" her entire life is evident. Nini Ferguson, a fellow horsewoman, recalled the limitless energy displayed by the Queen at the Windsor Horse Show in 2001. Aged 75, Elizabeth was as nimble as ever, following Philip as he competed in a carriage-driving marathon. "She drove her own Range Rover to each of the obstacles every half mile," said Ferguson. "She would watch him do the obstacles, then run back and jump in the car. She was in her wellies, with her scarf flying, followed by four or five corgis. She had such spirit and energy, and she seemed so young."

---

* "I have walked myself into my best thoughts, and I know of no thought so burdensome that one cannot walk away from it," said Danish philosopher Søren Kierkegaard. Triggering the body's relaxation response through its rhythmic, repetitive motions, walking, unsurprisingly, was the one activity Prince William intuitively turned to immediately after the death of his mother. For "the first two days" after the tragedy, says biographer Penny Junor, "he went for long, long walks alone" in the Scottish countryside.

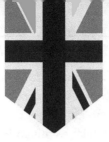

TWEEDY MODE

OR RULE #11—DON'T BRING
HEELS TO BALMORAL

When duty calls me I must go,
To stand and face another foe.
But part of me will always stray,
Over the hills and far away.

—ENGLISH FOLK SONG

iguratively speaking, the House of Windsor is turned inside out, like an inverted onion. The further you go inside the royal circle, the farther you must go—quite literally—outside. Country life and outdoor pursuits are so deeply embedded in the Queen's heart, they almost function, for her, like the mythical Scales of Anubis. Souls who wish to rise in her assessment are generally judged not by their glamour, celebrity, university degrees or impressive knowledge of world affairs, but by their fondness (or fear of) fresh air and good clean dirt. If you're not keen on sliding into a pair of wellies and trudging through damp moorlands or crawling across hillsides on your stomach to track an elusive deer, if you don't fancy picking up dead birds during grouse-shooting season (and putting dying specimens out of their misery with a firm whack) or hand-plucking a few fleas off your trusty hunting dog, then you better find yourself another royal family. You will be weighed and found sadly wanting by the Windsors.

Princess Diana, for one, never quite passed this trial by nature. Though she entered the family seemingly enthusiastic about country pursuits, it was little more than a temporary flirtation. Once married to Prince Charles, Diana had no intention of squelching about the muddy countryside or standing alongside her husband to angle for salmon in chilly rivers. Watching the outdoorsy highland games in Braemar, Scotland—an annual tradition for the royals—was an unmitigated bore for Diana. Cosmopolitan to her core, she failed to find the amusement in "grown men trying to throw telegraph poles," a reference to the ancient Scottish sport of tossing the caber. The same proved true for Margaret Thatcher. Her absolute ineptitude for country life made any real connection with the Queen virtually impossible. As prime minister, Thatcher would stubbornly arrive for her September visit to Balmoral in high heels, ill-prepared for the simplest country walks with the Queen. "Does the prime minister like to walk in the hills?" inquired a guest, shortly after Thatcher's visit. "The hills? The hills?" returned Elizabeth. "She walks on the road!"

On the flip side, a natural outdoorsy temperament can make up for innumerable deficiencies in the Windsor camp. Enter Sarah Ferguson. Despite her Diana-like propensity for scandal, Sarah always enjoyed a closer daughter-in-law bond with the Queen because of their shared love of country activities. "The Queen and I both doted on horses and dogs, on farming and open air," said Sarah. Bonding with Elizabeth over a gallop made her feel "favored and blessed."

Camilla Parker Bowles didn't follow the rule book in the slightest either, but she made her slow-but-sure transformation into the Duchess of Cornwall largely due to the same trait. "I love to get my hands dirty," says Camilla, whose passion for being outdoors has ultimately made her hugely more compatible with the nature-loving Prince Charles than Diana ever was. And though the Queen took years to accept their extramarital reality, it's significant that when finally deciding to heal the rift in 2000, Elizabeth and Camilla were able to start the process over a chat about their mutual love of equestrian sports. From the Queen's perspective, few sins cannot be eventually pardoned if—after a long day in the fields—you are willing to smell, and oftentimes look, like a horse.*

In her memoir, Crawfie takes full credit for turning Elizabeth into the countrywoman we know today. "Until I came," she insisted, Princess Elizabeth "was never allowed to get dirty." All jaunts to the park involving strict adherence to the paths. Crawfie believed she shook things up a bit—"I started a few innovations"—filling Elizabeth's childhood with the joys of rolling about in grass and falling into slimy ponds. Crawfie was soon observing that "[Elizabeth] was never happier than when she was thoroughly busy and rather grubby." It's a great story of rogue governess versus the prim Palace establishment, but the truth, in this case, is more interesting.

✳

Elizabeth comes from a long Hanoverian line of sprack outdoorsmen—people who've always felt excessively more relaxed in a shabby tweed jacket than an ermine robe. George III spent so much time outside, traipsing through muddy fields to indulge his interests in all-things agriculture, his subjects fondly dubbed him "Farmer George." Queen Victoria positively delighted in catching borderline hypothermia on her beloved Scottish hills, and George VI loved to relax by pulling up weeds in the garden at Royal Lodge. So naturally, Elizabeth was already being climatized to the great outdoors from an early age. Wheeled outdoors while still in her pram, she soaked up the bracing Scottish air that Victoria and Albert had fallen in love with nearly 100 years before.**

* Though admittedly better looking, Catherine Middleton's transition into the royal family was similarly eased by her displays of outdoor energy. After her first visit to Balmoral, Charles was thrilled to discover that Catherine "is clearly a country girl," said an aide to the prince, "which is a huge advantage" in the royal family. "The Queen is going to like this one," predicted the Balmoral staff.

** Queen Victoria's notorious beliefs in the therapeutic benefits of cold moorland breezes began early, shortly after a near fatal illness as a teenager. Her physician at the time, Sir James Clark, recommended the princess "be as much in the open air, and in *healthy, bracing* air" as possible. She would later attribute her speedy recovery to his prescription, giving her, says historian Lucy Worsley, "a lifelong passion for fresh air and chilly temperatures." Apparently anything over 60 degrees Fahrenheit and she felt positively "dissolved."

Long before Crawfie came on the scene, it was a royal childhood sprin-kled with a healthy bit of dirt. As the Queen's cousin Margaret Rhodes recalls:

> We were raised to believe that it was positively immoral to stay indoors regardless of the weather. One had to get outside and do something useful: chop wood, make a bonfire, pull out ivy, weed the garden or go for a bracing walk. The children of a nearby family who lolled around all day reading magazines and novels were cited as exam-ples of degeneracy. To this day I feel guilty if I remain inside for any length of time.

On top of which, Elizabeth's childhood coincided with a national "nature" awakening of sorts. Influenced by such books as *The Secret Garden* (where characters make miraculous improvements in health by spending more time outdoors), British nannies religiously threw open nursey windows and took their charges for daily blasts in the crisp air. "Fresh air makes for healthy living," nannies in training were told. Boy Scout and Girl Guide troops were soon springing up all over Britain, providing the nation's children with a weekly outlet for reconnecting with nature.

Lured by the prospect of camping expeditions, pitching her own tent and cooking sausages over an open fire, Elizabeth joined the Girl Guides in 1937—providing a vivid reminder of what she, as an elev-en-year-old, most valued at the time. It certainly wasn't twirling about in a princess dress. Arguing to allow Margaret to join the troop as well, Elizabeth pointed out, "She is very strong, you know. Pull up your skirts, Margaret, and show Miss Synge [the Guide director].You can't say those aren't a very fine pair of hiking legs, Miss Synge. And she loves getting dirty, don't you, Margaret, and how she would love to cook sausages on sticks." Margaret eventually got in as a Brownie, and Eliz-abeth would look back on the whole adventurously messy experience with "fond memories."* Its lessons lasted for years after, especially the Guide-inspired habit of turning to nature as the healthiest outlet for the emotions. As a fellow Girl Guide put it, "There is nothing like chopping a hefty log to relieve one's feelings." The Queen's unswerving mental stability would owe it a great deal.

"For a woman who is constantly surrounded by people, the natural world has played a large part in keeping her sane," writes biographer Ingrid Seward. Even when she is far away from the expansive Scottish landscape at Balmoral or the endless fields around Sandringham, Elizabeth still needs daily, tangible connections with nature in order to recalibrate her mind. Just pulling up a few weeds in her garden or feeding the ducks and swans in the Buckingham Palace pond will suffice. Biographer Sally Bedell Smith calls it her "primal communion" with nature and "her principal [means of] escape." The same was true for the Queen Mother. Also raised with a hearty appreciation for the countryside, particularly for the Scottish topography around her childhood home of Glamis Castle, the Queen Mother was famous for always preferring to be outdoors rather than in. She was endlessly throwing *al fresco* luncheons and fishing in the frigid River Dee well into her eighties. She gathered "fresh strength from the everlasting hills," she said. "I think that if I couldn't occasionally rest the eye & the spirit by the glimpse of green fields or purple mountains, I would go stark staring mad."

*

Psychologists Rachel and Stephen Kaplan reached the same conclusion in the late 1980s, in their seminal treatise on the brain-nature connection. They held that a walk in the woods is more mentally restorative than the same stroll down a busy city street because of the "soft fascination" of

---

* Elizabeth still has no problem with dirt, or with life's less glamorous realities. Once when visiting her stables at Kingsclere, she sensed there was something wrong with the ventilation system (a potential hazard for horses, which are highly prone to respiratory infections). Blowing her nose into a handkerchief later that day, she shocked her trainer by showing him the dark, mucousy contents. "I had a feeling that i was incredibly dusty in there, and there was no air," she said.

nature. A trait less due to its quietness (nature can be pretty noise) than the fact that nature is incredibly "soft" on our attention. Given humanity's former intimacy with nature, we are cognitively most comfortable when processing the visual cues of the natural world—a leaf, a tree, a hill, a sunset. Such things feel mentally effortless to engage with. Which is why, despite being far more sensorially complex, a walk in nature will feel like a brain-vacation, whereas the same exercise in man-made environments will feel oddly fatiguing. Richard Taylor, a physicist who has studied the nature connection, believes "fractals" are at the bottom of it. The complex patterns seen in clouds, trees, flowers and snowflakes are, paradoxically, so easy on the human eye, simply looking at them, Taylor has found, can reduce our stress levels by as much as 60 percent. Or increase it, whenever we withdraw from these primal pick-me-ups.*

Significantly, the only moments in the Queen's life when she has truly *not felt herself* is when she has been nature deprived. In 2003, after tearing cartilage in her right knee, she uncharacteristically expressed her frustration to a friend, feeling oddly fidgety and weak from, as she said, "languishing indoors" after the surgery. It's Elizabeth's one and only gripe for the job she inherited. If she doesn't read fast enough, the daily-delivered red boxes could entirely detach her from the natural world outside her window. And on heavy days, Elizabeth admits, "I do rather begrudge some of the hours that I have to do [reading] instead of being outdoors."

Some prime ministers, like Margaret Thatcher, might view such escapades outdoors—trudging through the heather-clad hills of Balmoral—as a cold, wet, needless expenditure of time and energy. Or take the more befuddled view of Tony Blair, who called his

---

* Even our immune system is boosted when we break out more into nature, particularly among trees. "There is no medicine you can take that has such a direct influence on your health as a walk in a beautiful forest," says Dr. Qing Li, whose research has shown that simply breathing in forest air raises the body's natural level of killer cells, a type of white blood cell that powerfully fends off disease. Such findings have fueled Japan's widely popular "forest bathing" movement and might additionally explain why Elizabeth feels legitimately improved after a visit to the wood-speckled landscape of Balmoral, where there is "always the fresh wind-borne smell of pine" on the air, says biographer Sarah Bradford.

nature-packed "country house" weekend at Balmoral "a vivid combination of the intriguing, the surreal and the utterly freaky." But these public servants are in office for a very limited time and so can afford to coop themselves up in Downing Street if needs must. The Queen is in the job for life, however, and takes a more holistic approach to her basic human needs. She shares the philosophical long view of Sir John Lubbock: "To lie sometimes on the grass under the trees on a summer's day, listening to the murmur of water, or watching the clouds float across the blue sky, is by no means a waste of time." Arguably, the Queen would never have lasted so long without the coping mechanism of the countryside—a royal survival skill both she and Philip have passed on to their children.

All four of them developed a deep, appreciative knowledge of the wildlife around their Scottish and Norfolk country homes. Philip taught them how to fish in the peat-brown pools of the River Dee, and Elizabeth took them stalking for deer in the nearby hills, making sure their cheeks were ritually smeared with the blood from their first kill.* For a princess who had everything, Anne remembers that the real "pure luxury" of her childhood were the days spent galloping with her mother across "miles of stubble fields" or experiencing the "autumn colours of the rowans and silver birches, the majesty of the old Scots pines" around Balmoral. The beauty of nearby Lochnager bewitched Prince Charles to such a degree, he wrote a bedtime story for his younger brothers, "The Old Man of Lochnager"—a lighthearted prelude to his later involvement in serious conservation efforts. And though he has sometime taken his unbridled love for nature rather far, as only Charles can overdo it (once admitting that he talks to his garden vegetables to help them grow), no one can doubt his genuine passion. Straight out of George

---

* Contrary to the old reproach against the English upper classes—"What a fine day it is. Let us go out and kill something!"—there's an important conservational logic behind the practice of deer stalking. As the Queen's cousin Margaret Rhodes explains, "The natural habitat can only support a certain number of deer and once the grass and heather off which they feed is exhausted, they then die a slow and horrible death from starvation, which is why they have to be culled annually." Moreover, every bit and bob of the deer is either used in the royal kitchens or sold abroad, even down to its hooves and eyeballs.

III's playbook, Charles has gone on record stating that if he wasn't a prince, he would be a farmer.

Much to Diana's annoyance, William and Harry felt the pull of rural life as well. Based with the boys in London during the week, Diana tried enticing them with the metropolitan delights of fast-food chains, cinemas and amusement parks, but come the weekend, William and Harry couldn't wait to rush off to Charles's country estate/farm of Highgrove. The "boys adored it . . . after a week cooped up in Kensington Palace," says biographer Penny Junor. Highgrove was "the perfect environment for noisy, energetic and inquisitive small boys." There was soft, turfy spaces to break into a run, animals to ride and feed and chase, woods to explore and dusty haystacks to fall into. Diana rarely joined them at Highgrove and, when she did, would more often be found sequestered inside: chatting on the phone with friends, flipping through a magazine or watching a movie. She didn't understand the appeal of the countryside, or why young Prince William wanted to be a gamekeeper when he grew up. She was especially envious of the way William and Harry seemed to prefer their nanny "Tiggy's" recipe for fun, far and above the amusement of whooshing down a funnel slide with their mother while the press gleefully snapped their photograph. "I give them what they need at this state," said Tiggy with the wisdom of a surrogate Windsor: "fresh air, a rifle and a horse." But then again, neither did most of the country understand the Windsor way of thinking when Diana died. During the immediate aftermath of the accident, the Queen was widely attacked for "keeping" the boys at Balmoral. Yet she endured the mob-like hysteria for as long as possible, almost to the point of seriously rupturing the monarchy's public image, because she firmly believed in the power of nature to restore. And those few quiet days—buffeted by soothing brooks and the surrounding pine trees—worked a hidden healing the press could never understand. It was where the princes needed to be.

Perhaps Elizabeth had remembered the moment when her own world momentarily stopped, and nature, unbeknownst to her, saw fit to prepare her for the coming trial. It was an extraordinary case of royal destiny repeating itself. Just as her predecessor Elizabeth I heard the news that she had become Queen at the age of twenty-five while seated *under* a tree, Princess Elizabeth became Queen at the same age while *up* in a tree. During the early hours of February 6, 1952, while on a Commonwealth tour in Kenya, Elizabeth and Philip were sleeping overnight in a wooden hut nestled atop a giant fig tree and planning on waking early to watch the majestic wonder of an African dawn. Meanwhile, sometime in the night and across an entire continent, King George suddenly died in his sleep. Deep in the African wilderness and cut off from all communication, however, Elizabeth was virtually the last British citizen to learn that she now reigned over all of Britain, Northern Ireland and the Dominions beyond the Seas. A historic blessing in retrospect. Far more important were those last few precious hours of incubating rest within, quite literally, the leafy arms of nature.*

---

* Elizabeth's maternal grandfather, the Earl of Strathmore, would have been proud. By all accounts an enchantingly kind, soft-spoken gentleman, he was incredibly fond of trees and tenderly maintained the forests around his Scottish and English estates. Often mistaken for a common laborer with his old raincoat tied with a piece of twine, he was "so well versed in the lore of the seasons and the plants and beasts," says biographer Carolly Erickson, "that he almost seemed like a forest creature himself."

HIBERNATE

OR RULE #12—REST LIKE YOUR KINGDOM DEPENDS ON IT

Labor is a craft, but perfect rest is an art.
—ABRAHAM HESCHEL

The British monarchy knows what life without a little rest can do. Twice over now reckless princes have nearly destroyed it because they didn't know when to take a break. In the nineteenth century there was Prince Albert, a grinding workaholic who wedded Queen Victoria with big plans for reforming the country, and the royal family, in his own industrious image. One worthy project barely finished before he was working late into the night on the next, until he finally admitted to feeling "more dead than alive from overwork." Ignoring the pleas of his physicians, who identified concerning links between his rapidly failing health and his relentless work ethic, Albert would be truly *more dead* before his forty-third birthday. Victoria found it easier to blame the entirety of Britain for the premature loss (Albert could do no wrong), so she cut herself off, for years at a time, from the people Albert worked himself to death for. The fateful decision left a Queen-sized hole in the heart of the country, quickly filled by some of the strongest antimonarchical feelings the kingdom has ever seen. A century later, with a lamentable disregard for his own family history, Prince Charles inadvertently caused the same. His inability to put aside his ceaseless work to spend any quiet time with Diana was already breaking his marriage apart long before either of them looked for love elsewhere. Even on Christmas Day, Diana took second place to a stream of frenzied memos Charles dashed off to his staff, many of whom couldn't help but admit, with exhaustion, that, "he never, ever stops thinking, he never stops pursuing ideas." Diana was breathless with abandonment, setting off a chain of scandals that tore their lives apart and left her dangerously vulnerable, while the entire royal family teetered on the edge of massive public disapproval. To rephrase the old nursey rhyme: the kingdom was nearly lost, and all for the want of a few hours rest.*

This is not the time to juxtapose the Queen as some patron saint of rest and relaxation. As we have already seen, she has worked just as tirelessly as Charles and far longer than Prince Albert (by about fifty years). But she has clearly worked smarter: putting a little more value on what both men refused to make time for. With her typical use of measured understatements, Elizabeth simply professes that "it's nice to hibernate for a bit when one leads such a moveable life." She knows the public wouldn't be amused by a Queen who jaunts off for workfree holidays— however much they enjoy and demand such downtime themselves—so Elizabeth has never made much of it. Not so much from false modesty, but because her "holidays" have never been remotely workfree . . . and presumably she doesn't want to brag. Parliamentary paper work, prime ministers and those ubiquitous red boxes are no respecters of vacation time when you're the Queen. As an adult, Elizabeth has never had a genuine holiday on the beach or traveled anywhere overseas purely for a bit of fun in the sun. Her "tours" abroad have all been work-away trips, carefully engineered by her government to provide some ulterior service to the country. But she seems okay with that. More than okay, as a matter of fact. "Sunbathing," says royal writer Brian Hoey, "is the last thing on her mind."

---

* Charles doesn't seem to have learned the lesson very well. In her first official interview as Duchess of Cornwall, Camilla spoke openly about her husband's all-engrossing work habit: "He never, ever stops working. He's exhausting . . . I am hopping up and down and saying, 'Darling, do you think we could have a bit of, you know, peace and quiet, enjoy ourselves together?' But he always has to finish something."

How Elizabeth *prefers* to rest is intimately entwined with her personality. She may have shaken more hands than anyone in history, but she is, at heart, far more introverted than people realize. "The world's most famous introvert," according to *Reader's Digest*. And introverts recharge very, very differently than extroverts. Outgoing with a natural bias for stimulating environments, extroverts might think a crazy week in the Caribbean, zip-lining and mixing with the locals over a bonging steel drum, is the epitome of holiday decompression, but it would just about level an introvert's energy. Because introverts only truly rejuvenate when the stimulation dial is turned considerably down. Hence a true vacation, by introvert standards, means ample time for quiet, circumspection, seclusion, calming rituals and, apart from a few trusted companions, privacy. To inherit a role that has left her, as it were, on the wrong side of the extroverted tracks (where there is as much privacy, said Princess Margaret, "as a goldfish in a bowl"), to be a truly effective Queen, Elizabeth has always needed to routinely reconnect with her inner introvert.*

Her annual pilgrimage to Balmoral is therefore vital to her overall well-being. Unlike her other country estate at Sandringham, where she spends Christmas and New Year, and which is intersected by a busy network of public roads, Balmoral is a veritable bubble of royal privacy. Public roads go around, not through, the 50,000-acre Scottish estate, creating a level of isolation that, while boring Princess Diana to tears (a true extrovert), the Queen finds inexpressibly peaceful. "You can go out for miles and never see anybody," said Elizabeth once, with a marked tone of relief. Many forget that Balmoral literally represented peace during the early days of World War II. Both Elizabeth and Margaret were safely sequestered there for the first few months of the conflict, far removed from the dangers of London where their parents were resolutely holding the fort at Buckingham Palace. "Lights were going out all over Europe," their governess recalled, but "up there in the

---

* If you're uncertain where you personally fall on the introvert/extrovert scale, it's easiest to begin with this classic question: Do you feel energized by a night out with friends or do you feel oddly drained, as if you need some quiet time afterward to recuperate? If you fall somewhere in the middle, you might be an *ambivert* (equal parts of both), in which case, hearty congratulations—you can fluidly enjoy the best of both personality worlds.

Highlands all was peace. . . . There was no bombing up there." Today, though the Queen continues to work every day of her eight-week stay at Balmoral—receiving daily bombshells of news from her government—it is principally alone-time work, which for an introvert is still regarded as a restoratively "hibernating" experience.*

※

In her best-selling treatise on what makes introverts tick, aptly named *Quiet*, Susan Cain posits that some of the world's most creative and productive people have relied on similar hibernation periods to excel in their work. Introverts like Charles Darwin shamelessly turned down dinner parties and went on long, solitary walks in order to better incubate his ideas. So too did Theodor Geisel (better known as Dr. Seuss) who, despite his effervescent literary persona, rarely met his fans and needed hours of alone time to fuel his imagination, preferring to work in a hermit-like bell tower outside his home in California. "Solitude matters," says Susan Cain. "For some people it is the air that they breath."

The insensitive, hyper-extroverted British press has never understood its tremendous importance, especially in 1997. While still smarting from Diana's death, a frenzied rush to "modernize" the monarchy included demands that the Royal Yacht *Britannia* be decommissioned, after over 40 years of service to the Crown. It was an ill-judged move in retrospect. Not only did it ignore *Britannia*'s vital function as a floating diplomatic office, allowing the Queen, as head of state, to visit remote parts of the

---

* Luckily, Elizabeth has never equated rest with sofa-slouching inactivity. "The very idea of a vacation doing nothing is abhorrent to her," writes Brian Hoey, which further explains why a seaside getaway lounging endlessly at the shoreline has never appealed to the Queen. As a girl she became restless, typically after 30 minutes, during periods of forced relaxation in the schoolroom. And Elizabeth still prefers to "rest" by doing some playful activity she enjoys, often outside and usually involving horses. The practice is sometimes called "deliberate rest" today, and psychologists like Mihaly Csikszentmihalyi believe it to be far more rejuvenating than simply reclining on your back, explaining that "hobbies that demand skill, habits that set goals and limits, personal interests, and especially inner discipline help to make leisure what it is supposed to be—a chance for *re-creation*."

Commonwealth she would never have been able to reach, it ignored its dual role as a royal sanctuary where the Queen, for a few treasured days each year, could experience a level of privacy her subjects daily take for granted. More cozy than opulent inside, visitors remarked on the "homeliness" of the yacht "which fits in with the Queen's personality. It's not a grand place." But Elizabeth, as ever, graciously bowed to the latest whims of shortsighted politicians and gave it up, only shedding a few tears at the decommissioning ceremony—one of the rare moments Elizabeth has cried in public. The tears weren't for a mere ship, as the press blindly liked to believe; they were for the precious solitude and the cherished family memories it represented. Which could explain why other monarchies throughout Europe—including the Danish, Spanish and Norwegian—have ignored their critics and wisely kept hold of their own royal yachts.

As someone who originally backed the building of *Britannia*—partly to give the overworked King George VI a well-deserved break—Winston Churchill was no stranger to the critics of rest himself. As First Lord of the Admiralty during World War I, Churchill got into the habit of taking afternoon naps to revive his energy and sharpen his wits. Though he constantly had to justify its importance to others, for at least an hour in the afternoon, he was strictly unavailable for government meetings. It became "one of the inflexible rules of Mr. Churchill's daily routine that he should not miss this rest," said his private valet Frank Sawyers. Even in the War Rooms, the underground labyrinth below London where the top secret complexities of World War II were orchestrated, Churchill would retire to a special room to get his forty winks. He likely could never have embodied the indefatigable wartime spirit of Keep Calm and Carry On if he did not take time to calmly recharge himself. "Nature," he argued, "had not intended mankind to work from eight in the morning until midnight without the refreshment of blessed oblivion which, even if it only lasts twenty minutes, is sufficient to renew all the vital forces."

Expertly captured in the film *Darkest Hour*, Churchill must further defend these daily rest periods to George VI, a borderline workaholic who is baffled by the prime minister's inability to bend his seemingly juvenile napping rule, especially during the war. The poignancy of the exchange, of course, is that the work-exhausted King would be dead in little more than a decade while Churchill (who smoked just as heavily and drank much more) lived to 90, guiding Elizabeth through her most vulnerable early years as Queen. The lesson was clearly internalized. When the writers of *The Servant Queen and the King She Serves* received Elizabeth's rare permission to capture her tireless contributions to British society as she neared her ninetieth birthday, they made sure to include the equally important reminder of how it has all been possible: "She takes her holidays . . . She doesn't justify her existence by how hard she works or feel that the world cannot go on without her. There is a time to rest."

Think Like a Queen

When the odds are hopeless, when all seems to be lost,
then is the time to be calm, to make a show of authority.

—Ian Fleming, *On Her Majesty's Secret Service*

The London Summer Olympics committee had, perhaps, the most unenviable task of 2012. Attempting to capture the essence of every icon of Britishness for the Opening Ceremony—from the NHS to Harry Potter—the millennia-old monarchy must have proved an especially sticky wicket. Specifically, how does one get to the nub of a Queen that represents an entire nation in a way that would be instantly understood by millions of diverse viewers in less than five minutes flat? What they ultimately decided on—holding their breath for Her Majesty's approval—would be the closest they came to perfection. Elizabeth would cameo in a short James Bond sequence, opposite actor Daniel Craig, saying far more *through* the role than her one opening line of "Good evening, Mr. Bond." Her performance exuded calm: from the moment Bond enters her office (presumably rescuing her from an impending threat), to the nonchalant way she boards the helicopter, to her ultimate plunge over the Olympic stadium in a Union Jack parachute (via a stunt double). It was all played exquisitely with an absolutely unruffled "needs must" expression on the Queen's face. And it sent the stadium's spectators, once they recovered from their disbelief, into uproarious cheers of approval, led by shouts of "Go, Granny!" from William and Harry, who were just as surprised by the performance as the rest of the country. Because for all the Bond-style fun, every Brit knew that it wasn't really a performance at all. This *was* the calm Queen they knew and admired: someone more likely to take one for Team Britain, even if it meant theoretically parachuting over London, than to ever make an emotional fuss.

Long ago, Elizabeth appears to have settled on "serenity" as her most identifiable regal trait, and every biographer since has been hard-pressed to find even one moment when she has broken character. To Ingrid Seward: "She is the most reliable, unflappable, least complaining monarch in history." To Andrew Marr: "She has uttered not a single shocking phrase in public. There are no reliable recorded incidents of the Queen losing her temper, using bad language, or refusing to carry out a duty expected of her." Elizabeth has been shot at, repeatedly charged by angry horses, conversed with a suicidal madman who broke into her bedroom, bore the hurling rocks of Irish protestors, faced down a rogue cricket ball which nearly lopped off her head and endured it all with a level of self-composure and courage that mystifies her bravest coworkers. In the case of the rogue cricket ball, as it zoomed into the stands and crashed into an adjacent seat, sending everyone else jumping to their feet, Elizabeth stayed seated, *cool as a cucumber*, to use a phrase now practically synonymous with the Queen herself. "I never saw her scared in any way," admits Edward Ford, her assistant private secretary for fifteen years. Even the impressive imagination of children's writer Roald Dahl couldn't imagine Elizabeth as anything but cool and emotionally collected. In the *BFG*, when the titular giant makes a startling appearance outside Buckingham Palace, only the Queen keeps calm: "She didn't scream as the maid had done. Queens are too self-controlled for that. . . . Considering she was meeting a giant for the first time in her life, the Queen remained astonishingly self-composed."

Iconic traits have a way of being iconically misunderstood. Some believe, for instance, that Elizabeth's composure is an effortless by-product of her position—that the only big secret behind her inner tranquility is "never having to look for a parking place," or so joked John Julius Cooper, the 2nd Viscount Norwich. Others think she was simply born this way, pointing to treacly accounts from her infanthood by royal admirers who peered into her cradle and saw "the sweetest air of complete serenity" on baby Elizabeth's face . . . and no doubt a golden halo too. Either way, it isn't generally assumed that the Queen has worked for the characteristic that has largely come to define her legacy. But she *has* worked for it, and it is a *learned* ability: the ability, as her friend Monty Roberts observed, "to get calmer in the face of problems rather than allowing herself to get her adrenaline up and to panic." The only problem being, Elizabeth has made it look too easy, deftly hiding the years of practice and the sound philosophical strategies she has purposefully embraced for long-term survival.* And though they might come second nature to her today, they haven't, by any means, come as naturally as people might think. As it is, we see only the serene result. But don't be fooled, explains Prince William, a man after the Queen's calm heart. "We're like sort of ducks," he says, "very calm on the surface with little feet going under the water." Paddles and patterns we'll explore in the following pages . . .

---

* A fitting nod to that survival: the Queen has lived through every transition of James Bond actors onscreen and, moreover, was crowned in the same year the first Bond book was released, 1953.

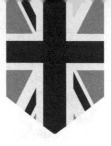

THE MERRY STOICS
OF WINDSOR

OR RULE #13—JUST GET ON WITH IT

CHURCHILL: *The duty which has befallen you . . .*
is the greatest honour on earth.
ELIZABETH: *I might struggle, on occasion, with that honour.*
CHURCHILL: *Just never show that struggle, ma'am.*
It's not what your subjects want from you.

—PETER MORGAN, *THE AUDIENCE*

Death looked like Diana's ultimate revenge. At least for one bizarre week in 1997. Spending the last years of her life extolling the exhilarating highs of emotional openness—bearing her full-frontal heart to any reporter who would listen—Diana left the world by seemingly splintering into a million carbon copies. Everyone now had permission to be a drama princess too, and Britain let lachrymosely loose on a scale never witnessed before. Judgments were passed, tears were counted like currency and people's characters were measured by how deeply they felt Diana's passing, regardless of whether or not they personally knew or liked her. Tony Blair (like a true politician) gave the emotive mob what it wanted. He quivered his voice on cue and spoke passionately of the "people's princess" as if they were lifetime pals. But the Queen held firm. Apart from a few historic concessions (including flying the Union Jack at half-mast over Buckingham Palace and speaking directly to the country "as a grandmother"), she had no intention of taking part in the national weep-a-thon. Public displays of grief had never been her style, and she wasn't going to start now. The decision left the media seeing revolutionary red. If the Queen didn't get in touch with her inner emotional crazy lady, the *Daily Express* warned, the monarchy's imminent demise would come "a giant step closer." Other headlines screamed, "Show Us You Care," failing to understand that it was precisely due to the Queen's profound care that she showed such stoic reserve. To manufacture a good blub, just because it was temporarily fashionable, would not only have been in defiance of who she is, it would have perilously undermined who her country has always needed her to be.

Specifically, monarchy is not so much a shoulder to sob on but a strong back to lean against. For Winston Churchill, it was one of the "inestimable services" the Queen rendered to the country. "Above the ebb and flow of party strife," he observed, "the rise and fall of Ministers and individuals, the changes of public opinion or public fortune, the British monarchy presides, ancient, calm and supreme within its functions." Becoming a royal rock for her people has necessitated a level of quiet, self-contained dignity that, in an age where celebrities splatter us with every emotional detail of their lives and reality stars cry at the drop of a rose, is both astonishing and refreshing. Her deeper emotional life and her personal political opinions remain, to this day, a complete mystery. The Queen met with Margaret Thatcher every week for eleven years but has never revealed what she personally thought about her. The same goes for every one of her fourteen prime ministers. Elizabeth's personal views on the controversial Suez Crisis of 1956 and the recent Iraq War are likewise absolutely unknown. For the job and for the country, said former Foreign Secretary David Owen, Elizabeth has had the "courage to be boring." Viewers of Netflix's *The Crown* have already noticed the pattern. As the series progresses, Elizabeth (the character) is getting fewer and fewer main story lines of her own. The real Elizabeth has simply been too good at hiding her private feelings, and thereby avoiding scandals, that the writers of the show have needed to look elsewhere for royals gone naughty. It might make for less sensational drama, but it has certainly created a stronger monarchy.

*

Emotions have simply never served the House of Windsor well. Consider the recent rise and rapid fall of Meghan Markle's royal career. A true scion of Hollywood culture, where actors are cheered for being emotionally "real" and vulnerable, Meghan played her part as Duchess of Sussex using the same celebrity script. Her audible complaints about the toughness of the job and overemphasizing her zeal for environmental politics were admittedly slight, but more than enough to make her sound whiney, pampered and elitely hypocritical (especially when she used a fuel-guzzling private jet for summer holidays). She broke the two cardinal rules laid down by the Queen Mother many years ago—"never complain, never explain"—and generated such antipathy in the press that Prince Harry was forced into semi-abdication in order to end the blistering attacks.* But Meghan was by no means a targeted anomaly, as much as she likes to think so. Royal history is one long sob story of individuals who chose emotional release over reserve and lived to regret it. In the heat of his exploding rift with Diana, Prince Charles thought the touchy-feely world was ready for *his* side of the emotive story. He thought woefully wrong. *Prince of Wales: A Biography* was widely ridiculed and did more self-inflicted damage to his image than Diana could have gleefully wished for. The ghost of Mary, Queen of Scots, was still alive and well. In 1587, her unmanageable fiery temper found her without a kingdom, a crown or a head to rest it on. Emotionally incapable of restraint, she joined the hotheaded-turned-beheaded ranks of Anne Boleyn and, later, King Charles I.

From the earliest age possible, therefore, Elizabeth was inculcated with the belief that her survival, in more ways than one, depended on the ability to control her emotions. There was nothing austere or

---

* In contrast, Kate Middleton's emotional discretion has proven to be her ultimate royal security. She has been "utterly discreet," writes biographer Penny Junor, despite being "hounded and harassed and followed and photographed; she has put up with jokes about her middle-class origins . . . and criticized for not having a proper job. And never [has] she risen to the bait, confided in anyone outside her family, or put a foot wrong."

repressive about Elizabeth's childhood, as we have seen, but she was "brought up," says her first cousin Mary Clayton, "to be in control of [her] temper and moods, and never allow [her] moods to dominate." Whether it was a scraped knee or a sad parting from her parents as they left on a royal tour, her main goal was to quickly recover and, above all, to never "make a fuss"—especially within earshot of a reporter. "I've been trained since childhood never to show emotion in public," says the Queen. It was an honest, preemptive effort to curb what many viewed as the scourge of past sovereigns. Known as the "Hanoverian temperament" or the "Hanoverian spleen," the descendants of George I appeared to have a genetic propensity for incredibly bad moods. Like his petulant father and grandfather before him, George VI had temper tantrums (as an adult) of such hellish magnitude, they took on the notorious name of "gnashes" among his family and staff. "He was not an easy man to know or to handle," admitted his equerry, James Stuart. Expensive furnishings, on occasion, had to be removed from his presence lest he destroy a priceless antique.* A dispositional hand-me-down bequeathed to Prince Charles, who's been reported to fly into rages when he can't part his hair neatly, or smash a friend's country house window when he wanted fresh air, or rip a porcelain sink from the wall after a fight with Diana.

And though it seems unthinkably out of character for her today, the Queen entered the world with a fair bit of Hanoverian hotness under the collar too. According to her governess, Princess Elizabeth could lash out at Margaret with a determined "left hook" and once decided—"goaded by boredom to violent measures"—to rebel against an infuriating French teacher by tipping an entire bottle of writing ink on her own head. Eruptions which were soon minimized and tamed by her mother's calm and soothing example, long before the public knew of any other version of her temperament. Waving her parents

---

* George's "gnashes" were generally calmed by the sympathetic wit and pragmatism of his wife. During a particularly infuriating tour of South Africa, hoping to convince the country's increasingly hostile Nationalists to remain in the Commonwealth, George gnashed out to his wife, "I'd like to shoot them all!" To which she quietly replied, "But Bertie, you can't shoot them *all*."

off at the dockside as they departed for a propaganda tour of North America, just before the outbreak of World War II, Elizabeth was already instructing Margaret on the finer points of royal restraint. The handkerchief Margaret was holding was for one purpose, Elizabeth told her: "To wave, not to cry."

Admittedly difficult to appreciate in our let-it-all-hang-out century, emotional reserve was an ideal which seeped through the whole of British society at the time. This, after all, was the reign of the stiff upper lip: a roughly hundred-year period between the 1870s to the mid-1960s when the majority of Britons seemed to unanimously agree that, when it came to the public expression of feelings, it was far better to restrain than to release. It was, as Helen Mirren remembers, "the noble generation," or as the psychologist Mihaly Csikszentmihalyi has argued, one of the formative moments in human history when "people were held responsible for keeping a tight rein on their emotions" (comparable to ancient Sparta, Confucian China and Republican Rome). Elizabeth grew up during its apogee. "It was a different world," recalls George Harewood, another royal cousin. "People kept much more private and much more quiet [about personal matters]." The screenwriter for *The Queen*, Peter Morgan, saw it as such a fundamental key to Elizabeth's personality, he developed much of his award-winning film around the stark contrast between her quiet dignity in the wake of Diana's death to the "narcissism and intolerance of pain of our generation." A generation which is more likely to snicker at than understand the now legendary displays of inner grit in Britain's recent past—like the unknown soldier who, when lying wounded in a muddy trench on the Somme, was said to mutter only a "mustn't grumble" in consigned bravery.* But as biographer Gyles Brandreth entreats, "The stiff upper lip wasn't a joke: it was a much-vaunted

---

* British culture historian Sarah Lyall points to the vivid contrast displayed by David Beckham in 2003 after a tussle with his coach in the Manchester United locker room, when a kicked shoe accidentally collided with Beckham's forehead. "Rather than taking it on the chin," says Lyall, he "scraped his highlighted hair back into a girly headband and strode into the path of the waiting flashbulbs. He made sure the photographers got a good shot of his forehead with its sad injury and its reproachful Band-Aid. He spread around the story that the wound had needed stitches."

national characteristic." Moreover, it was largely influenced by one of the most ancient and practical mental strategies ever devised: Stoicism.

＊

Often confused with the emotionally constipated character of Spock from *Star Trek*, Stoicism the philosophy (founded in Athens around 301 BC) did not promote the annihilation of all emotions, only minimizing the negative ones. Among the first thoughtful psychologists of the ancient world, Stoics argued that the good life was one based on the daily pursuit of *ataraxia*, "tranquility of mind." Not "a zombie-like state" of emotional oblivion, explains philosophy professor William B. Irvine, "Stoic tranquility was a psychological state marked by the absence of negative emotions, such as grief, anger, and anxiety, and the presence of positive emotions, such as joy." Above all, the Stoics believed that people were intrinsically resilient and rational beings: whatever circumstances befall us, we could always choose our emotional response. As modern Stoic Ryan Holiday clarifies, "real strength lies in the *control* . . . the *domestication* of one's emotions, not in pretending they don't exist."

Over two thousand years later, Stoic philosophy (via the British stiff upper lip) would be tested *en masse* and found to be an incredibly effective technique for coping with some of the most traumatic moments of the twentieth century. At the outbreak of World War II, British psychologists feared that mental hospitals would be overrun with an influx of new patients mentally crippled by the horrors of war. The public simply wouldn't be able to cope with, what would be, shell shock on a massive scale. Ordinary Brits proved them totally wrong. Emotional resilience was the norm, not the exception, and there was no uptick in the occurrence of mental illness during the war. Like the Queen Mother, people truly believed that Churchill's famous battle cry—"Never Flinch, Never Weary, Never Despair"—was the best way to survive hardships. They saw nothing helpful in analyzing negative emotions or raking over distressing memories from the past. Far better to just "get on with it," as the wartime slogan went. BBC broadcaster Bruce Belfrage kept calmly reading the 9:00 p.m. news bulletin on October 15, 1940, despite a bomb crashing into the Broadcasting House seven floors above him, covering him in dust and soot. Stoicism kept him chugging along. Though nothing came close to the stoic success story after the horrific Aberfan disaster of 1966. When a deadly landslide buried a village school in Wales (along with 116 children and 28 adults), the parents and surviving children of the community were not descended on by grief counselors or well-meaning therapists, nor did they claim victim status or "closure" by demanding compensation for their loss. By all modern assessments, without professional help, the villagers should have been mentally crushed under the grief they faced on their own. As it turned out, they coped heroically. School was resumed two weeks later. A year after the tragedy, child and family psychologists were amazed by how normal and adjusted the community appeared. "The villagers had done admirably in rehabilitating themselves with very little help," reported *The Times*.*

Respect for private grief was so strong in those days, Elizabeth didn't immediately rush to visit the scene of the tragedy. How could more invasive cameras and newsmen truly have helped the village in its suffering? It was a mark of true sensitivity, which she intuitively repeated on the death of Diana. Her subjects, of course, had moved on since then, preferring a hypersensitive session on their therapist's couch—taking offense and casting blame at everyone but themselves—to their grandparents' self-reliance and stiff upper lip. But the Windsors had not. They are truly the last of the legendary Stoics.

*

The only time the Queen has uttered the slightest trace of a public grumble was in 1992, in her famous "Annus Horribilis" speech. It capped the end of a relentlessly horrible year for the monarchy, which witnessed the eruptive separation of Charles and Diana, the separation of Andrew

---

* How they pulled through might additionally lie in what sociologists identity as our current "victimhood culture" versus the more prevalent "dignity culture" at the time. In a flourishing "dignity culture," people are generally viewed as emotionally sound, self-reliant agents who are able to cope with personal struggles in their own time and way, without needing input from professionals or someone/something to place therapeutic blame upon. Prince Charles demonstrated this cultural shift to victimhood in *The Prince of Wales: A Biography*, wherein he blamed his personal failures on his upbringing, his parents and his boarding school. Typical therapy lingo, but it garnered him next to no public sympathy.

and Sarah Ferguson, the divorce of Princess Anne, a devastating fire at Windsor Castle, and an angry public refusing to finance its rebuilding. "Few of us are likely to experience such a high level of family distress in one year, and very few of us will ever have the added pressure of seeing it all made globally public," says royal writer Mark Greene. The Queen, however, used only the briefest of British understatements to remark on the events that would have crushed someone more emotionally brittle. "1992 is not a year on which I shall look back with undiluted pleasure," she said. It was a perversely positive way of assessing the situation, but it is the only way the Queen knows how to move on, and move on quickly, from personal tragedies she can do nothing about. And it's evident that the future King, Prince William, has watched and learned.

As someone who has endured more than his fair share of adolescent trauma—his parent's media maelstrom of a divorce, their dual admittance of adultery on television, his mother's death, his father's mistress becomes part of the family—it's interesting to note which emotional path William has decided to follow. After all, he had a mother who pioneered the reality-star right of self-expression, priding herself on leading "from the heart, not the head." A child of the post-Stoic era, Diana "preferred talking to repressing, sharing her pain to keeping it to herself, having her own way to ceding to others," says culture historian Sarah Lyall. And when the famous opportunity came to spill her emotional innards on BBC's *Panorama* program, Diana leapt on the cutting board, divulging everything from her own infidelities to her eating disorder, as a strange new breed of cannibalistic viewers licked it up.

But such overexposure of private sorrows embarrassed William, who saw firsthand that it didn't bring his mother any cathartic relief or lasting happiness.* In comparison, his grandmother's practical stoicism in the face of equal hardships must have seemed like an oasis of calm. It was an obvious choice. "He's taken a leaf out of [Elizabeth's] book," said Miguel Head, William's long-standing private secretary. And though William is careful not to use the now therapeutically unfashionable terms of "stoicism" or "stiff upper lip," he has long been a true Stoic in all but name. He is described, by the people who know him best, as "a

---

* We'll explore why in the next rule.

steady bloke, unemotional and unflappable . . . he doesn't get massively excited about stuff." Sandy Henney, Charles's press secretary, who spent more time than most around William during his formative years, says he rarely allowed himself to be emotionally exposed, a trait she found, after Diana's addiction to oversharing, to be incredibly refreshing. "I think he has an innate sense of self-protection," says Henney. "If you ask him a personal question he will be as honest as he wants to be, but you will never get down, thank God, into the real root of William."

Biographer Penny Junor refers to it as William's "psychological armour": how he has managed to come through heartrending trauma by not giving too much of his real heart away. And though you might think such stoic reserve would isolate William from a world whose collective hankie has long since gone soggy, it has done the opposite. William is now universally regarded as one of the most likable, dependable, relatable and well-adjusted royals in the Windsor arsenal. As one of his friends perfectly expressed it, "He's someone you'd like to have alongside you in the trenches."

Evidently Queen Mary was mistaken. Way back in 1913 she feared that emotional "finesse" had all but disappeared from the modern world, with garish unrestraint taking its place. Britain was going to the weeping dogs. But nothing has really changed. We still gravitate to individuals like Elizabeth and William who exemplify Stoic virtues and cannot help but ostracize others, like Meghan Markle, who reflect a level of vulnerability we don't actually want to see in ourselves. Our culture's truest heroes (not necessarily televised talent show winners) remain stoic figures, like Nelson Mandela and Mahatma Gandhi, who overcame extraordinary adversity, not by opening up their psyches for all to see, but by truly just "getting on with it." We still very much have what Roman moral philosophers called *nobilitas animi*, "nobility of mind or soul," a magnetism towards emotional, almost regal dignity deeply embedded in our conscience, whether we're born royal or not.*

---

* Prime examples: Rudyard Kipling's "If" poem, epically infused with Stoic ideals, is still frequently voted Britain's number one poem (it was also a particular favorite of Queen Mary's). Ditto the 1946 British film *Brief Encounter*, a love story which applauds emotional restraint; it was still being named the most romantic movie ever made in 2013.

"The Britons of this generation [are] as strong as any," said the Queen, reassuring her subjects during the 2020 coronavirus outbreak. "The attributes of self-discipline, of quiet good-humoured resolve...still characterise this country."

Polls taken a year after Diana's death offer a fascinating perspective on this. Despite the media-generated hype that Britons had universally thrown off their Stoic shackles to embrace their inner teary-eyed princess, 50 percent of the public thought their fellow subjects had stupendously overreacted while over 70 percent charged the media with overblowing the entire episode. Rather, what most people look back on with patriotic pride wasn't Elton John's melodramatic rendering of "Candle in the Wind" or Earl Spencer's finger-pointing eulogy, but something far more intrinsically noble. It was the poignant image of Prince William and Harry displaying an inner strength the assembled, tear-weary crowds desperately needed to see—both of them walking courageously behind their mother's coffin *not crying*.

OSTRICHING

OR RULE #14—THIS THRONE
AIN'T BIG ENOUGH FOR NEGATIVITY

Don't be defeatist, dear. It's very middle class.
—THE DOWAGER COUNTESS, *DOWNTON ABBEY*

When God made the Queen Mother, it must have been in a Teflon factory. Scandals that stuck like calcified cheese to other Windsors were, to her, but piffling crumbs to be daintily swept away. The affectionate grandmother of the nation, and about as controversial as a newborn babe fresh from the maternity ward, the Queen Mother was uniquely off bounds to a critical press that would cuff their own grannies if the story paid enough. *Except* when it came to her most iconic mental quirk. Then eyes started rolling and politely padded claws came out. The Queen Mother was a regal Pollyanna, they said. She buffered herself inside a bubble of optimism and spoke of life as if she were living in a P. G. Wodehouse novel, where everything was sure to turn out *tickety-boo, old bean, what ho*! She was outdated, out of touch—a real "imperial ostrich" who all-out ignored negativity like it wasn't even there. Pessimists were decidedly ticked off. Even biographer Craig Brown couldn't speak of her singular "pursuit of happiness" without getting in a slight jab. The Queen Mother might have achieved "perpetual radiance," he conceded, but she did so "by ring-fencing herself from anything unpleasant." Her critics have clearly been suffering from a classic case of royal myopia, a forest for the trees scenario. Preoccupied by scoffing at what the imperial ostrich was avoiding, people failed to see everything she gained.

In fact, necessity was the mother of optimism in her case. Although generally buoyant, the Queen Mother had a marked tendency to brood, especially after emotional shocks, which could spiral her into crippling depressions. The trauma of the 1936 abdication crisis ostensibly laid her up in bed with the "flu" (of the psychological sort) that left her, she said, "groping in the darkness of disillusionment" and "overcome with misery." She was "very depressed and miserable," she confided to a close friend. It was a brief, but concerning, period of almost complete neglect of her royal duties. Such a reclusive episode, as the new King's consort, could not be allowed to happen again. Like Victoria before her, she knew the country would tolerate almost anything in a queen— except weakness. Recognizing that negativity acted like a "vampire" on her psyche, which "drained away something of the joy of living," she adopted the ebulliently positive attitude that would become her trademark—and more crucially, her means of mental survival during World War II. "I am still just as frightened of bombs & guns going off," she told a cousin as explosions rocked London, "in fact I'm a beastly coward but I do believe that a lot of people are, so I don't mind! . . . Tinkety tonk old fruit, & down with the Nazis."

Such displays of cheeriness would prove contagious. Visiting the war-wounded and stumbling through the devastated rubble of the Blitz, her plucky optimism, her perpetual smile, her tireless encouragement to "keep the old flag flying. Hooray," made her a unifying symbol of Britain's indomitable spirit, oftentimes in the face of hopeless odds. Hitler is thought to have grudgingly dubbed her "the most dangerous woman in Europe" for her extraordinary ability to keep the free world's emotional morale up. It was an unsought role for a self-proclaimed "beastly coward" who found it only human to crumple under negative pressure and "so much easier to yell & pull down & criticize, than to restrain, & build, & think right." But she was now part of a new breed of British royalty: Kings and Queens who forfeited their hard-won power of regal authority for the "soft power" of kindness, empathy, and always looking for the good. She was now officially in "the happiness business," to quote Martin Charteris. And the Queen Mother did more than accept the duty; she internalized it.

Her emotional comfort zone, even in private, became an echo chamber of the biblical passage "whatever is noble, whatever is right, whatever is pure, whatever is lovely, whatever is admirable . . . think about such things." Like Julie Andrews romping on a downy bed in *The Sound of Music*, the Queen Mother could fill entire letters describing "all the things I like"—"fairies and owls, and bluebells & Americans . . . fat butlers, porters, the smell of tangerines . . . a good tune, lovely colours, French accents, puppies, bath salts, & a million more." But for the seamier side of life, she adopted the strict policy of "least said soonest mended." As biographer Elizabeth Longford explains, "Temperamentally she was too much amused by life to weigh up its every conundrum with painstaking deliberation, or to waste the buoyant hours on analysing problems that could be dealt with more naturally by charm and empathy." Even the ghost of the abdication crisis was rarely allowed to rear its negative head. By all rights, she could have endlessly ranted against the Duke and Duchess of Windsor, who selfishly dumped "this intolerable honour" on her family's lap, but her closest niece and lady-in-waiting, Margaret Rhodes, recalled, "not once in all the years I was with my aunt—not once—did I ever hear her say anything remotely unpleasant about them." A proclivity for the positive that only increased as she got older. Mildness marked her every response, even during the IRA terrorist bombings of the 1990s when the royal family was target number one. Her most heated pronouncement on the crazed bombers amounted to, "Oh, they really are very naughty and very, very confused." To some, such astonishing aplomb in the face of real danger only solidified her "ostrich" image. To others, it reinforced her reassuring role as the unflappable "mum" of the nation. Major Colin Burgess, her equerry during the nineties, was of the latter opinion. "The Queen Mother," he said, "reminded me of the colonel in *Apocalypse Now* walking along the beach, with explosions going off all around." A strategic legacy she has undeniably passed down to her daughter.

Elizabeth's head isn't (and cannot be) as fully buried in the sands of positivity as her mother's—her job throws up a virtual treadmill of unignorable irritations—but she has nevertheless gone "ostrich" as much as possible too.* Like her mother, Elizabeth "became adept at blocking dangerous questions or simply avoiding 'unwise' subjects," says Andrew Marr. The Queen heartily dislikes confrontation, if she can avoid it, and will choose silence over an emotional flare-up if ever disappointed by a family member or staff. Her worst verbal bombshells, if they surface at all, haven't been known to extend any further than the mild "well, that was a fair-to-average stupid thing to do." She doesn't find pleasure or relief in pouring out her woes to sympathetic listeners, vastly preferring the technique she learned from the "imperial ostrich" herself: "I find that I can often put things out of my mind which are disagreeable," Elizabeth told a friend.

Philosophically, it all sounds like a juvenile riff on the classic tale of royal make-believe *A Little Princess*, by Frances Hodgson Burnett. "When things are horrible—just horrible," says perpetual-optimist Sara Crewe, "I think as hard as ever I can of being a princess. I say to myself, 'I am a princess, and I am a fairy one, and because I am a fairy nothing can hurt me or make me uncomfortable.'" Cute, but rather delusional for the rest of us, no? Downright dangerous even. We've been taught that examining our negative feelings is cathartic, self-caring and unquestionably healthy (particularly if it's "assisted" by a mental health professional) and that trying to suppress troublesome thoughts or conquer them or—heaven forbid—"bottle them up" is one nervous twitch away from going all-out bonkers in a mattress-lined room. As such, we might still ostensibly wish Elizabeth "happy and glorious" whenever we sing *God Save the Queen*, but we do so with a little less therapeutic conviction these days. Perhaps releasing a bit of Palace ennui and pent-up anger—ideally at Meghan and Harry—would be good for her also? At any rate, how could it possibly hurt? Quite a massively concerning bit, as it turns out.

＊

As recent research into negativity, resilience and neurology has shown, there is nothing unanimously liberating about having a good weekly

---

* In a delightful case of serendipitous symbolism, there are ostrich feathers stuck into the Tudor cap of Elizabeth's Order of the Garter regalia, one of her most historically important vestments.

cry in your therapist's office. Neither is the almost universally accepted doctrine that "uninhibited emotional openness is essential to mental health," asserts psychiatrists Sally Satel and philosopher Christina Hoff Sommers, who have recently teamed up to study the pitfalls of modern therapy culture. "For many temperaments," they argue, "an excessive focus on introspection and self-disclosure is [actually] depressing. Victims of loss and tragedy differ widely in their reactions: Some benefit from therapeutic intervention; most do not and should not be coerced by mental health professionals into emotionally correct responses. Trauma and grief counselors have erred massively in this direction."* The promise of greater mental clarity through an intense plunge into painful memories is usually just a Freudian pipe dream—and a very narrow one at that. Studies have shown that negativity drastically reduces our brains' emotional range of vision. The more we ruminate over troubling thoughts, the more we "impose a lens that shows a distorted, narrow view of our world," said psychology professor Susan Nolen-Hoeksema of Yale University. Being introspective and too analytical about sadness is only a shortcut to more sadness, she explains, giving our brains "greater access to sad thoughts and memories" and making us "more likely to interpret [past and future] events in a sad way." Coping becomes more difficult, not less, and can, she warns, "take you down paths to hopelessness, self-hate, and immobility."

When researchers studied the emotional aftershock experienced by parents whose children had died of sudden infant death syndrome, the results refuted the common assumption that *talking through* the pain is cathartic. The parents who consciously followed the modern precepts of grief therapy—who consciously endeavored to think about and make sense of their loss—were more emotionally raw eighteen months later than the parents who didn't attempt to therapeutically work through the

---

* Sarah Ferguson's exchange with celebrity therapist Dr. Phil typifies the error. The calm way Sarah recounted her mother's death, via a car crash in 1998, bothered Dr. Phil, who found it too composed for comfort: "You just told me a horrifying, tragic end to your mother's life, and you told me about it as though you were ordering lunch," he said. Despite the fact that the tragedy occurred over ten years prior and Sarah believed—rightly so—that she had mentally healed from the event, Dr. Phil quickly pronounced her "emotionally bankrupt."

tragedy but instead moved through it naturally on their own. Similar findings have been replicated over a diverse range of grieving individuals, including abused women, Holocaust survivors and the surviving partners of AIDS victims. Indeed there is vast scientific support behind the Queen Mother's stoic suspicions that "some things are best not discussed."

In 1981 when Elizabeth was fired upon during Trooping the Colour ceremony (whilst sitting vulnerably sidesaddle on a horse), her iconic "even keel" barely wobbled. Nor did she feel the need to emotionally dredge up the incident later that night when Prince Edward telephoned her from school. She didn't even mention it. To mentally replay the fear and confusion of the day would have been counterproductive— or as the Queen Mother liked to say, "unhelpful"—in her attempts to move forward. All of this could be easily misconstrued as *being in denial* or *delaying grief* when, in truth, Elizabeth is what psychologists more accurately term a "purposeful repressor." Compared to ruminators (people who repeatedly reflect over distressing events), repressors seemingly break all the rules of our modern mental health culture. They spend very little time talking about, let alone acknowledging, negative events and will quickly exchange a passing unpleasant thought for something more optimistic. Yet far from being mentally maladjusted or out of touch with the real world, studies have shown that repressors are actually more popular among peers, perform better at solving problems and enjoy a healthier self-image than their ruminating counterparts.* Likewise, heart attack patients who confront their recent health scare with a repressive coping style have been found to have higher levels of psychological well-being and less anxiety months later than non-repressors who suffered the same severity of attack. "We must learn not to hold our hurts and waste our time crying, like children who've bumped

---

* "The moods of repressed people may be more balanced," concluded a team of psychological researchers in a report called "Is Repression Adaptive?" Their study divided a group of high school students by their coping styles: repressors (who subdued troubling thoughts), sensitizers (who paid close attention to their emotional state) and intermediates. The repressors were rated, by their peers and teachers alike, as more successful both academically and socially than the other two groups. They were also rated as having greater frustration tolerance and self-worth.

themselves," instructed Plato in *The Republic* over two millennia ago, "but to train our mind to banish grief by curing our hurts . . . as soon as it can."

＊

Every year, for over six decades now, the Queen attempts to impart a little repressive wisdom of her own. Her annual Christmas broadcast rarely touches on the slightest chord of negativity, however turbulent the past year has been for the nation or for her personally. Throughout the 1970s, when Elizabeth experienced the crushing loss of four close members of the family and the acid breakdown of Princess Margaret's marriage to the Earl of Snowdon, she never referenced the personal pain to her subjects, always preferring to niggle out the good instead. "Perhaps we make too much of what is wrong and too little of what is right," Elizabeth remarked near the end of 1974, a particularly gloomy year for Britain as a whole. But that was the "trouble with gloom," she said, with astonishingly accurate insight. "Gloom . . . feeds upon itself and depression causes more depression."

Though we assume the smartest people are "in touch" with the fouler feelings of life, being too introspective can become "the psychological equivalent of picking at the scab on a wound," says philosophy professor William B. Irvine. Doing so "can delay the natural healing process." Sometimes permanently. Princess Diana's emotional wreckage of a psyche offers a somber example. A natural ruminator fueled by the "feel it to heal it" pseudo-philosophy of the twentieth century, Diana spent years (and a small fortune) bouncing from one tear-soaked therapy session to the next. Already privately addicted to probing her past for painful memories, she went through several psychotherapists, tried Jungian dream analysis, dabbled in hypnotherapy to visualize her angst by "throwing it up an imaginary chimney and burning it," and vented her rage into a therapist-supplied punching bag.* Diana even

---

* It's been recognized for well over half a century that anger catharsis or "anger release" therapy or simply "letting off steam" is hugely counterproductive, tending to increase, rather than decrease, feelings of rage. Back in 1959 psychologist R. Hornberger already observed that when people were allowed to "release" their emotional frustration (in this case, by pounding nails

tried colonic irrigation (basically a wet vacuum up her bum) in the hopes that it would "take all the aggro [aggression] out of me." But nothing delivered the mental breakthrough or self-actualizing freedom each treatment promised. Diana was "as unsure of herself at her death as when I first [met and] talked with her," recalled her friend Richard Kay. "I found in the end that therapy was pointless for me," Diana admitted mere months before she died, turning against a system she now recognized as keeping her in a vicious cycle of vulnerability. "Everyone knows how to treat you when you are vulnerable," she said. "But if you show any sign of strength, then it is they who end up feeling intimidated. And they try to squash you back to where you were." By then it was too late. As her biographer Sally Bedell Smith explains, Diana had already fully succumbed to "emotional hemophilia," being utterly unable to clot the flow of her negative feelings. The slightest psychological wound would gush forth such toxic quantities of tears that young Prince William, on one occasion, had to push tissues under the bathroom door she had locked herself behind. It was tragic evidence of the narrowing power of negativity. Just three years before her death, Diana was sitting in a group therapy session when she revealed the extent negativity had consumed her. Asked to focus on "something positive" that had happened to her in the previous week, Diana drew a complete blank.

Psychologist and grief expert Lucy Hone recognizes it as the simple, but vast, difference between why resilient people, like Elizabeth, manage to rise above tragedy while others, like Diana, tend to crumble. "Resilient people are really good at choosing *carefully* where they select their attention" and "make an intentional, deliberate, ongoing effort to tune into what's good in [their] world." The habit of looking for the positive in every circumstance (what psychologists call "benefit finding") is now identified by Hone as one of the universal "secrets of resilient people." Intimately acquainted with tragedy herself (when a car crash killed her twelve-year-old daughter), Hone says the vital skill set of benefit finding, giving herself permission to "accept the good" and dial down the negative,

into a willing object), they acted more aggressively after the fact than people who contained their frustration. Little over a decade later, the president of the American Psychological Association, Albert Bandura, called for a complete halt to all so-called *therapeutic* forms of "venting."

"saved me in my darkest days." Especially when she realized the power of one strategic question: Is indulging in this negative thought or behavior "helping or harming me?"—a truly self-caring query if there ever was one, and something which sounds remarkably similar to the Queen Mother's refusal to dabble in "unhelpful" topics of discussion.

Then again, no one made a more circuitous journey back to the bedrock of ostriching than Sarah Ferguson. Under the rather disconcerting self-advice of "free your mind and your bottom will follow," she traveled halfway around the world to discover a psychological wisdom that was, once upon a marriage to Prince Andrew, only a few doors down at Buckingham Palace. Writing in *Finding Sarah: A Duchess's Journey to Find Herself*, she recounts how a rough year of personal scandals, followed by borderline mental breakdowns, brought her to Thailand, where she emotionally collapsed at the feet of an Indian guru. His spiritually enlightened advice? Let go of "negative mind chatter," he told her. Specifically, picture negative thoughts as if they were "poop balloons" in the sky (I'm not making this up). "Yes," her guru insisted, "start visualizing those thoughts as balloons filled with poop. See them floating over your head. If you hold on to them, you'll puncture them with your fingernails, and get covered with poop. Let them go; watch them soar out of your sight. Out of sight, out of mind."*

Poor Sarah. She could have saved herself the plane fare (and an untold number of royal poop balloons) if she had, long ago, paid a little more attention to the emotional gurus of Windsor. As it was, she missed out on Martin Charteris's number one tip for survival, the invaluable advice he once imparted to every new recruit at the Palace: "Never forget you're in the happiness business." To forget it, frankly, is to really bury your head in the sand.

---

* Elizabeth Gilbert, author of *Eat, Pray, Love*, also found her inner ostrich by way of flying off to a third-world locale. Previously coping with "powerful sadness" through the debilitating "comfort of tears," her spiritual sojourn in India revealed a better way, as her own (more tactful) guru put it: "You should never give yourself a chance to fall apart because, when you do, it becomes a tendency and it happens over and over again. You must practice staying strong, instead." Gilbert began repeating the wisdom of repression "about 700 times a day: 'I will not harbor unhealthy thoughts anymore.'"

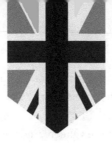

VIEW FROM ABOVE

OR RULE #15—THERE IS NO "I" IN MAJESTY

*She must be above everything . . . I feel very sure of this—
she must remain a serene and wise figure outside the ravings
& ramblings of this agitated world.*

—THE QUEEN MOTHER EXPLAINING ELIZABETH II'S POSITION

Every morning the Queen begins her day with a ritual that would ruin not just the morning but likely the entire month of someone with thinner skin. With the singular exception of the *Racing Post* (which she reads purely for fun), Elizabeth confronts an exhausting array of national newspapers, including the tabloids, laid out beside her breakfast table each morning. It's her dutiful way of staying plugged-in to the public mood, but it's also a darn good way to lose one's appetite. Seldom are the headlines splattered with anything but ulcer-generating reminders of what the Queen has done wrong, what any number of her family has done wrong, what her prime minister is too afraid to tell her or simply what a unscrupulous reporter has decided to entirely make up.* Most days, the Queen's breakfast table

---

* It's been rumored that during the early 1980s, the press office at Buckingham Palace attempted to keep a daily updated file of untrue stories about the royal family. The project was soon abandoned, writes royal historian William Shawcross, as "'it took up too much time.' And too much space, no doubt."

is a veritable buffet of tea, toast and media misery. Even Prince Philip, with his usual pachyderm exterior, can't stomach it. "I don't read the tabloids," he once admitted. "I glance at one. I reckon one's enough. I can't cope with them. But the Queen reads every bloody paper she can lay her hands on!" Curious behavior for an emotional ostrich like Elizabeth. More curious still when you consider the fact that none of this ceaseless attention has gone to her head.

She was barely out of diapers when it all started: *Time* put her on its cover in 1929, confirming her global celebrity at the whopping age of three. At the time, sightseers would peer through park railings, waiting for a glimpse of the princess as she toddled on afternoon walks with her nanny. But nothing surpassed the level of adulation and interest Elizabeth experienced when still in her twenties. She was internationally "adored . . . as much as Diana was, perhaps even more so," writes historian Gyles Brandreth. "In the late 1940s and early 1950s, in Britain, in France, in countries around the world, thousands—tens of thousands, sometimes hundreds of thousands—turned out to cheer her." But remarkably, Brandreth adds, Elizabeth "did not take it personally."

All displays of self-absorption had long since been eradicated from her personality. At seven years old and still figuring out the boundaries of royal power, Elizabeth was once greeted by the Lord Chamberlain with the casual, "Good morning, little lady." Either truly affronted or simply wishing to point out his titular error, Elizabeth replied with the haughty, "I'm not a little lady. I'm Princess Elizabeth!" Unfortunately, she said this within earshot of Queen Mary, who immediately marched her humbled granddaughter to the Lord Chamberlain's office for an apology. "This is Princess Elizabeth," began Queen Mary, "who one day hopes to be a lady." Elizabeth would never make such an imperious mistake again. Despite being next in line to one of the oldest thrones in Europe, she became admirably unaware of her own popularity, far more so than Margaret. Organizing their Christmas pantomime shows at Windsor Castle, Elizabeth was genuinely flummoxed at the high price Margaret wanted to charge for tickets. "Oh, you can't ask people to pay seven and sixpence. No one will pay that to look at *us!*" But Margaret knew a royal cash cow when she saw it. "Nonsense!" she said. "They'll pay anything to see us." Margaret would have made for a very different Queen. As it was, Britain got its least self-centered monarch in history. "Here we have the most famous woman in the world and yet she has never been remotely interested in fame," says journalist Lucy Draper. Elizabeth didn't feel the least desire to watch "herself" (via Helen Mirren's portrayal) in *The Queen*. "She cares not for celebrity, that's for sure," says Prince William, who knows his grandmother's bar of self-importance is set far lower than people generally assume.* When the glamorous divorcée Mrs. Tom Troubridge was about to join the British royal family in the 1970s, becoming Princess Michael of Kent (after dropping a few hints of her own royal pedigree, extending back to Charlemagne), the Queen concluded with magnificent self-deprecation, "She sounds much too grand for us."

To think otherwise, to inwardly bask in the glory of outward majesty, "could have been corroding," says Prince Philip, adding that however easy it would have been to "play to the gallery," both he and Elizabeth "took a conscious decision not to do that." They have seen too many bubbles of self-preoccupation burst around them. The very reason Elizabeth sits on the throne, and not her uncle, is because Edward VIII's narcissism caused him to blindly overestimate his own popularity. Prioritizing his celebrity version of happy-ever-after, he permanently lost the

* His great-grandmother, the Queen Mother, was exactly the same. Marrying Bertie and becoming Duchess of York in 1923 (the first modern commoner to break the royal barrier) barely inflated her ego. Asked by a friend how he should now address her, she replied, "I really don't know! It might be *anything*—you might try 'All Hail Duchess', that is an Alice in Wonderland sort of Duchess, or just 'Greetings' or 'What Ho, Duchess' or 'Say Dutch'—in fact you can please yourself." Sixty years later, nothing had changed. During a high-profile event in the 1980s, a bellowing announcer called for "three cheers for Her Royal Highness" (the Queen Mother was a "Majesty" not a "Highness"). Though when the mortified event coordinator began to apologize, she pooed it off with an "Oh, please don't worry one little bit. I haven't been a Royal Highness for over 50 years, it made me feel quite young again."

respect of his family, government and subjects who found it impossible to cheer a king who always put himself first.

*

Before she gave them real cause for grief, Princess Diana troubled Elizabeth and Philip for the same reason. Her dividing line between Crown and celebrity seemed to be dangerously blurred. Clues that Diana was joining the royal Firm for the wrong reasons were concerning, like her comments at the first picnic she attended at Balmoral when dating Prince Charles. As the sumptuous luncheon took form—the perfectly polished silverware, the table linen, the menu cards—Diana squealed, "Oh! This is the life for me! Where is the footman?" Charles's friends sounded the alarm, sensing that Diana had "fallen in love with an idea rather than an individual." The *idea* would certainly become her most memorable asset. She could "play to the gallery" like no other royal, maneuver the press with the expertise of a PR professional and knew how to drive international media stories from nothing more than a single well-photographed pose. But the idea was also her undoing. The daily fluctuations of fame, the coverage each newspaper devoted to her unfolding royal saga, became the rod by which she both measured and pummeled herself.

Diana was her own worst paparazzo, analyzing every story written about her, not for staying detachedly informed, like the Queen, but for fueling a self-devouring hunger she found difficult to satiate. Like a social-media addict obsessively totting up *likes*, "Diana got pulled into a process she found fascinating and terrifying," writes biographer Sally Bedell Smith. "She could sit for as long as an hour, exclaiming that the tabloids were trying to make her look awful, inviting compliments from staff members on the flattering shots and reassurance about other images that bothered her." She turned so far inward, her own self-image became dangerously, sometimes suicidally, warped. "I didn't like myself," she admitted, feeling increasingly trapped by a compulsion to "perform" to a press mob she once intimately courted. As Peter Conrad puts it in his study of the Narcissus myth, "the longer you look at yourself, the more estranged you are from what you see."

This was definitely *not* what the "me generation" promised to people like Diana, neither does it square with today's culture of self-hood, where ego-obsessed Kardashians are rewarded with unimaginable wealth, where multitudes vie for publicity with every conceivable "share" of their lives, where our most popular form of photograph is the "selfie," even if it deigns to include the faces of others. All quite predictable behavior, in fact, according to Abraham Maslow's classic psychological construct, the "hierarchy of needs" (which helped birth the me generation). In it, individuals striving for *authenticity* move upward through baser needs, like love and self-esteem, to reach "self-actualization"—the height of human fulfillment. In other words, per the founder of humanistic psychology, we become exponentially happier the more we turn inward. Similar to Diana, Sarah Ferguson was a ready convert of this new model of the universe, where every self is solipsistically self-orbiting. At one point, Sarah's secret to mental well-being involved repeating the mantra "I love myself more than I ever imagined possible and others love me too . . . twenty-five times a day." But few realize that later in life, Abraham Maslow changed his mind. Influenced by clearer thinkers, like Viktor Frankl, who believed such self-preoccupation was ultimately self-harming, Maslow modified his theory. "The fully developed (and very fortunate) human being working under the best conditions," he said, "tends to be motivated by values which transcends his *self*." Maslow identified these luckiest of souls as "transcenders"—people very similar to the Queen, as a matter of fact.

✳

Elizabeth's entire reign has been a self-transcendent one. She has been a "lesson of modesty," writes political commentator Andrew Marr, especially in a world where "being oneself" has been proffered as "the highest human good." Elizabeth has always been "the opposite of Diana," says a former courtier. "She is the least self-obsessed person you have ever met. She doesn't think it is interesting to talk about herself." Even in the realms of grammar, the Queen is far more comfortable using the impersonal pronoun "one" than the more self-directing "I" or "me." It is almost as if she was viewing life events from a detached vantage point, from the outside in, as it were.* This is especially true when Elizabeth is compelled to make a boast, like when she remarked on her impressive record of absolute discretion during weekly talks with her prime ministers, saying, "They [prime ministers] know that *one* can be impartial . . . I think it's rather nice to feel that *one's* a sort of sponge and everybody can come and tell *one* things" (my italics). You could say Elizabeth is practicing what philosopher Pierre Hadot once termed a "View from Above" approach to life, practically the exact opposite of Maslow's original "hierarchy of needs" theory. It was, at one time, a widespread belief among Stoic philosophers, that the more you panned out from yourself—the more you considered daily events from a detached perspective, as if you were looking down on them from *on high*—putting those events into proper perspective and coping with the stress would be much easier. The Stoic Roman emperor Marcus Aurelius found he could think most clearly about the daily burdens of fame, military conflicts and ruling a rebelling empire by mentally distancing himself from the action, oftentimes by visualizing the events from the serenity of outer space.** "Survey the circling stars as though yourself were in mid-course with them," he exhorts. "Visions of this kind purge away the dross of our earth-bound life." The Queen Mother famously

---

* Closely related is the "majestic plural" or "royal we," a monarch's prerogative to speak of themselves in the third person, predating Elizabeth I and immortalized in Victoria's imperial put-down "We are not amused." It still comes in handy for the Queen today, as the embodied head of a very pluralized nation. Though sadly, no one else can get away with its usage without appearing certifiably bonkers. Like Margaret Thatcher who, in a Freudian-slip of imagined grandeur, frightfully confused the public when she regally announced, "We are a grandmother" after the birth of her first grandchild.

** Interestingly, this is one of the symbolic reminders of the Sovereign's Orb used in British coronations. The golden globe signifies the cosmic "View from Above" that all good earthly rulers should have, a reminder that monarchy itself is a "light above politics," says philosopher Roger Scruton, "which shines down on the human bustle from a calmer and more exalted sphere." Though it bears pointing out, just for clarity, that this is not the same "View from Above" espoused by Princess Pauline, Napoleon Bonaparte's shockingly haughty sister who, and I do not jest, liked to periodically use her servants as footstools.

mastered the art. Rather than internalizing slights or taking things too personally, she always strived for "placid detachment," says Major Colin Burgess. "If something did upset her," he recalls, "you never heard her say, 'Oh, I'm sad.'" Instead, she would use the impersonal modifier, "'Isn't it sad.'" The same was true for personal annoyances and disappointments: "'Oh, isn't that annoying?'" she would say, always carefully avoiding the internalities of me's and I's. "She took a detached view of virtually everything," Burgess noted.

*

Science has come a long way from Maslow's misguided theory of self-absorption to recognizing the virtues of "self-distancing." Getting out of our own heads turns out to be the easiest way for those heads to think clearly. Emotionally raw college students from Columbia University were among the first to confirm it. In a study that enlisted students fresh from a serious social rejection that left them with "overwhelming feelings of anger and hostility," researchers asked half the students to recall the experience through their own eyes and try to make sense of their feelings from an inward "self-immersive" perspective. The other half were asked to recall the experience too, but this time "from the perspective of a fly on the wall." Results from the two groups couldn't have been more strikingly dissimilar. The self-immersed group behaved as if they were reliving all the emotional pain of the experience. They felt as angry and hurt as if the event had just happened. The fly-on-the-wall group, however, completely reappraised the event. Their detached perspective allowed for clarity and emotional closure: for understanding why the painful event happened in the first place and for greater empathy both towards themselves and for the other party involved. Subsequent studies have revealed even more. Self-distancers have been found to have lower blood pressure, use more constructive strategies for solving problems and be more adaptive in negative circumstances.*

---

* Self-distancing has become a major feature of CBT (cognitive behavioral therapy), arguably one of the most effective treatments for severe depression and anxiety. CBT therapists try to help their clients put distance between themselves and their feelings, to understand that their self-immersed thoughts are just their individual (and oftentimes very distorted) interpretation

Like her or loathe her, self-distancing is arguably how Camilla mentally survived her own media firestorm. Once touted as "evil Camilla," blamed for breaking up the Diana-Charles fairy tale, not too many people could have endured the label "most hated woman in Britain" and live to become, years later, a respectable Duchess. But Camilla did so by getting out of her head as much as possible. "I was always brought up to get on with life and not sit in a corner and weep and wail," she explains. During the height of Diana's attempts to massacre her image, Camilla simply played along with self-deprecating humor. Knowing Diana's nickname for her, Camilla began answering the telephone with "Rottweiler here." Or catching sight of yet another ugly photograph of herself in the tabloids, she would simply yawn, "Thirteen double chins as usual." The responses were right out of the Queen's own playbook. Elizabeth has long known she doesn't always photograph well, that her natural baseline expression tends to fall into a Muppet-like frown "she herself has likened to Miss Piggy," says Andrew Marr. Yet rather than agonize over the fact, the Queen has chosen to become a detached observer of the amusement. When finally getting a chance to rewatch Charles and Diana's lavish wedding on television in 1981, Elizabeth caught a glimpse of her unintentional scowl in the front row. "Oh Philip, do look!" she chuckled. "I've got my Miss Piggy face on!" A brilliant testament to the accuracy of Iris Murdoch's philosophical hunch: "Happiness is a matter of one's most ordinary everyday mode of consciousness being busy and lively and unconcerned with self."

---

of reality, "not revelations of absolute truths that can be seen only one way," says psychologist Walter Mischel.

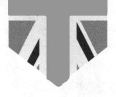

STINKING WILLIE

OR RULE #16—LAUGH WHEN
YOU WANT TO CRY

Oh look, Margo's on fire!
—Elizabeth II, a tad amused, when Princess Margaret's
hair accidentally brushed against a candle at a dinner party

H enry VIII had it much easier. He employed a full-time Groom of the Stool to deal with the literal poop of life (charged with the *privilege*, so to speak, of passing the King a flannel "to wipe his nether end"). Six centuries later, Elizabeth must apparently make do with a Stinking Willie. To quickly explain, before your imagination runs afoul: Stinking Willie is the name of a noxious Scottish weed found around the Balmoral estate that Elizabeth has taken to pulling up, by the vigorous handful, when royal poop happens. To some, weeding appears to be her only means of tension relief on days when "the Crown," as she herself has admitted, "does get rather heavy." For every *annus horribilis* the Queen has publicly faced, there are untold numbers of *dies horribilis*, horrible days, she privately endures. Yet she has more than garden weeds at her disposal. There are two tactics, specifically, the Queen has found to be incredibly useful for bouncing back from the nether end of monarchial drama, two reactionary strategies she has constantly come back to when life gives her a Stinking Willie. Starting with her personal favorite: humor.

The coping mechanism of comedy has an illustrious history among British royalty. Once personified by the acting court comedian, or King's "fool," the injection of levity into the monarch's life was once deemed so vital, the Office of the Revels was established in the late-medieval period to guarantee it. Jesters were often the only ones who felt safe enough to speak truth to power when trouble or scandal rocked the court. Their brand of humor was hardly sophisticated. Some of Henry II's jesters were only required to exhibit the triune talents of "a leap, a whistle, and a fart." But they were essential, nonetheless. The silly antics of Elizabeth I's court comedian, Richard Tarlton, famed for putting on mock duels with the Queen's little dog, was said to have "cured her melancholy better than all her physicians" combined.

The Windsors have kept, at least the heart of, the tradition alive. Becoming their own pocket jesters, they have trained themselves to search for the humor when things don't go according to royal plans. Take the incident in 1977 atop Snow Hill in Windsor Great Park. Elizabeth was *supposed* to light the first ceremonial bonfire that would signal a chain of beacons to be lit around the British Isles, marking her twenty-fifth year on the throne. Before she could set the bonfire ablaze, however, a fumbling soldier hit the emergency ignition switch, setting off an unintended chain of technical mishaps. "Your Majesty, I'm afraid everything that could possibly go wrong is going wrong," said the event coordinator, ready for a right royal smackdown. Instead, a glorious grin broke over the Queen's face. "Oh good. What fun!" she replied. Spotting the ridiculous in public, then having a good laugh about it in private, is sometimes "the only thing that keeps them sane," says biographer Brian Hoey. "If they didn't laugh privately at some of the antics they are forced to witness with outward solemnity, they would cry." An almost verbatim echo of Seneca's philosophic maxim, tendered two thousand years ago: "Laughter, and a lot of it, is the right response to the things which drive us to tears!"* The humor reflex is so institutional throughout the

---

* Stoics like Seneca recognized humor as one of the quickest ways to defuse stressful situations (undermining the modern misconception of Stoics as stone-faced killjoys). Cato the Younger found humor invaluable for staying tranquil when he was publicly insulted, particularly when a loudmouthed orator named Lentulus spit in his face. "I will swear to anyone, Lentulus,"

Windsor Firm, an officer aboard the Queen's former yacht, *Britannia*, said he once had to ask new recruits only two interview questions to determine their suitability for royal service: "Have you got a prison record; and have you got a sense of humor? And if they laughed at the first, there wasn't any need for the second."

Prince Philip effortlessly glided into Elizabeth's affection for much the same reason. Never taking himself too seriously, he donned a kilt on his first visit to Balmoral and, overcompensating for the embarrassment (which would become his hallmark), performed a mock curtsey in front of the King, doing any medieval jester proud. The King wasn't altogether impressed, but it clearly amused Philip's future wife, who would come to depend on his impromptu injections of fun. After mentally exhausting days on tour, Philip came to the rescue with a range of practical jokes, from setting off booby-trapped cans of nuts to chasing Elizabeth down train corridors with a horrific set of false teeth. For the Queen, his quick wit has always been priceless on painfully tedious days, though he has admittedly played the courtly "fool" a bit *too well* on occasion. A comedic specialty he has cringingly coined "dontopedalogy," or "the science of opening your mouth and putting your foot in it." His gaffable zingers have become so numerous and unsparingly broad in their offense, entire books are devoted to the curated "Philipism." Like the time he met the singer Tom Jones and asked, "What do you gargle with, pebbles?" Or to a driving instructor in whisky-loving Scotland, "How do you keep the natives off the booze long enough to get them through the test?" Or to an Australian Aborigine, "Still throwing spears?" Or, perhaps most famous of all, remarking on a dubiously installed electric fuse box, "It looks as though it was put in by an Indian"—one of the few gaffes he felt the need to correct with, if you please, another gaffe: "I meant to say

---

Cato calmly replied, wiping the spit away, "that people are wrong to say that you cannot use your mouth!" Today, cognitive behavioral therapists essentially use the same technique. Clients who are plagued by anxiety and negative thoughts are asked to imagine their doomsaying visions spoken in the voice of a funny cartoon character, like Daffy Duck or Elmer Fudd. "It may sound silly," writes psychologists Jonathan Haidt, "but it can quickly turn an anxious or upsetting moment into a humorous one."

cowboys. I just got my cowboys and Indians mixed up."*

Elizabeth could have done with a few less Philipisms over the years, but she wouldn't be the same Queen without them either. Philip's humor, said Martin Charteris, "has done the state some service"—proving invaluable for keeping Elizabeth's spirits up and, as an introvert, for making her social life much more bearable. It's a "common sight at parties," says biographer Gyles Brandreth, the Queen will be "chatting quietly with someone while Philip is at the center of a small group, laughing, entertaining his guests, telling a funny story. This has been going on for more than half a century. She makes intelligent, interested small talk . . . He keeps the party going."

Not to say that the Queen can't hold her comedic own. Philip might be the public jester, but Elizabeth can be "extremely funny in private," says former Archbishop of Canterbury Dr. Rowan Williams. A born mimic, she can have her family in stitches with her impersonations of British regional accents (her Yorkshire accent, apparently, can bring down the Palace). But it's her terse one-liners that have become her comic trademark: "It looks very damp," she said, on a visit to Niagara Falls in Canada. "I myself prefer my New Zealand eggs for breakfast," she remarked, after being in the firing line of an egg-throwing protestor in New Zealand. And the more confidentially witty: "Please tell the band under no circumstances to play excerpts from *The King and I*," before a state visit from the king and queen of Thailand.** She doesn't dare risk any more, as an un-regal attack of the giggles is often percolating just

---

* This is fun, let's continue: To a resident of the Cayman Island, "Aren't most of you descended from pirates?" To a group of British exchange students studying in China, "If you stay here much longer you'll all be slitty-eyed." To a policewoman wearing a bullet-proof vest, "You look like a suicide bomber." To NASA employees, on past moon missions, "It seems to me that it's the best way of wasting money that I know of." To British designer Stephen Judge, on his rather small goatee, "Well, you didn't design your beard too well, did you?"

** And my personal favorite: Touring the Jamestown settlement in Virginia in 2007, the Queen was shown various archeological discoveries, including an iron spatula-like implement once used "for severe constipation." Calling her traveling physician over, Elizabeth pointed to the rusty contraption and said, "You should have some things like that!"

below the surface. "I've seen the Queen laugh till the tears ran down her face," said a relative. She must therefore take preventative measures, especially on formal occasions, compensating with a tight-lipped expression that makes her look, as one cabinet minister has put it, "like an angry thunder-cloud." In actuality, she is often simply suppressing a laugh. On one occasion in the 1960s, when four ministers had badly bungled their first meeting with the Queen—kneeling on the wrong side of the room and awkwardly knocking a book off a table—Elizabeth looked "blackly furious" as she quietly bent to pick it up. Later, their superior returned to apologize, only to be stunned by the Queen's broad smile and admission of, "You know, I nearly laughed." It was then he realized that quietness was just another one of her useful royal strategics: "When she looked terribly angry it was merely because she was trying to stop herself laughing."

＊

Which nicely brings us to the Queen's second reactionary reflex: silence. If anyone alive has lived by the universal mom rule *If you don't have anything nice to say, don't say anything at all*, Elizabeth earns top marks. Though in her case, the mom rule would also include anything remotely political, nationally sensitive or internationally iffy. As journalist Deborah Orr has surmised, "Elizabeth appears to have applied the same logic to her reign as I did to my French O-grade [oral exams], which was deciding that the less I said, the less likely I was to make an error. It's an excellent strategy." What often gets wrongly attributed to shyness is, in fact, one of her longest-running preservation tactics. The Queen is "reticent," not shy, insists her biographer Elizabeth Longford, pointing out the important difference: "Reticence has its own good reasons for silence." In a world of perpetually open ears, where the slightest utterance can be twisted beyond any recognition of its original intent (just as Meghan Markle), tactical reticence has proved, time and again, the safest haven for royalty. A century ago, Queen Mary ushered the modern Windsors into a secular vow of silence, and the smart ones have stayed put.*

---

* If Queen Mary only knew she lived in accordance with Mahatma Gandhi's reported advice:

Elizabeth has elevated silence into an art form, becoming, as culture historian Peter Conrad puts it, "an expert semiotician, a transmitter of speaking looks." A glance, a nuanced expression can instantly communicate her pleasure or disdain. Politicians and courtiers know there can be a wide range of direct meanings in her "icy silence," says Andrew Marr, including "the 'you may go now' silence, the 'I disagree' silence and the plain 'you make the running' silence." Then there is what Paddington bear might call the Queen's "hard stare"—reserved for the soon-to-be-exiled oaf who has said something inappropriate or highly disagreeable in her presence. An eyewitness of *the stare* reports, "She never argues, she just looks at the person very blankly. The corners of her mouth don't turn down. It's not a hostile look, it's just a complete blank—and it's devastating." Constantine II, Greece's former king, considered the stare a crucial "talent"—"the capacity," he said, "of older European royals to look people in the eye and show them with one look that they have gone too far. My grandmother Olga froze out a group of Bolsheviks when they tried to seize her house during the Russian revolution. . . . The Queen has it too."

These are rare moments of royal displeasure, however, and by and large, the Queen's tactful capacity for quietness and her ability to listen, rather than speak (a rarity in our modern world), has comforted far more people than it has put off. Prime ministers especially. To unburden themselves to someone, perhaps the only one in the country, who will never publicly turn their words against them, who keeps no record of the conversation and who has no ulterior motive but to listen and ask thoughtful questions, can be incredibly therapeutic. Bystanders would observe Winston Churchill leaving his private talks with the Queen

---

"Speak only if it improves upon the silence." She didn't like the man, but followed his maxim to a tee. Especially during the regrettable moment in 1947, when surveying Elizabeth and Philip's wedding presents, Queen Mary came across Gandhi's unique contribution—a simple piece of linen he had woven himself. To her, it looked disgustingly akin to one of his loin-cloths (probably used) and therefore the height of bad taste. Prince Philip disagreed, but rather than publicly debate the matter, "Queen Mary moved on in silence," said a bystander. She was laying the groundwork, notes Elizabeth Longford, of "royalty's time-honored method of dealing with an awkward situation": silence.

positively "purring." Prime Minister James Callaghan also left "feeling marvelously refreshed," according to biographer Ann Morrow, and John Major described his weekly audience with Elizabeth as something akin to a session "on the psychiatrist's couch."

In large measure, this has been the Queen's social brilliance, especially when talking with ordinary folks. Great listeners tend to exponentially rise in the esteem of great talkers. Hence people generally emerge from a chat with Elizabeth praising her charm and effortless wit when, in reality, it is they who have done most of the talking. "If this is a strangely passive record of achievement," writes Andrew Marr, the passivity has been purposeful and carefully calculated, adding, "one has only to think of what trouble an activist, opinionated monarch might have got into during the 1960s, or the Thatcher years, or when New Labour was going to war in the Middle East." The Queen has a word for the tactic—"considered inaction"—borrowed from Walter Bagehot's famously forward-thinking advice for British monarchs in 1867. "Probably in most cases," he wrote, "the greatest wisdom of a constitutional king will show itself in well considered inaction." In other words, the smartest reactions are routinely marked not by public posturing, but by patience and restraint. Time alone can heal far more than any knee-jerk response, retaliation or gratuitous explanation.* British advertising guru Hugh Salmon sees it as the biggest takeaway of the Queen's career. "If you are in a position of leadership," says Salmon, "perhaps you should say less than you do. You do not have to justify your every decision . . . You have no need to impress. Or preach. Just get on with your job, set

---

* The Stoics referred to the strategy as *sustine et abstine*, "bear and forbear," a wisdom once widely imparted to British children. "Remember the two nice bears, bear and forbear," nannies would say, attempting to defuse nursery conflicts. The strategy is still very much applicable today, argues the modern Stoic Ryan Holiday. "Sometimes we need to . . . take some action," he says, "but we also have to be ready to see that *restraint* might be the best action for us to take. Sometimes in your life you need to have patience—wait for temporary obstacles to fizzle out. . . . Sometimes a problem needs *less* of you—fewer people period—and not more." The Russians, he cites, expertly used the strategy, defeating both Napoleon and the Nazis "not by rigidly protecting their borders but by retreating into the interior [of Russia] and leaving the winter to do their work on the enemy."

yourself the highest professional and personal standards, stand by them for the whole of your life and, while doing so, keep your mouth shut." One can only imagine the peaceful world in which all celebrities and politicians kept a little more royally mum too—taking time, as Shakespeare would say, to make "much ado about nothing."

Love Like a Queen

My crown is in my heart, not on my head.

—WILLIAM SHAKESPEARE

For a surprisingly large number of her subjects, the Queen pops in on a regular basis, usually at night, rather like Santa. Dreams about the Queen are so delightfully ubiquitous, at least one-third of all Britons are believed to routinely enjoy the pleasure. The settings vary, but the commonalities are marvelous: Elizabeth is often wearing a crown, tea is typically involved, the dreamer invariably demonstrates profound common sense that impresses the Queen (prompting the royals to wonder where the dreamer has been all their lives) and there's almost always the parting, pre-wake-up appreciation that Elizabeth is a very kind, lovable old lady indeed. Even nutcases who take their private dreams a bit further—oh, say, like breaking into the Queen's bedroom for an early morning chat—reach the same comfy conclusion. Michael Fagan, who committed that whopper of an indiscretion in 1982, walked away from the hostage-like encounter thinking the Queen was "a really nice woman." In the minds, hearts and nocturnal hallucinations of millions, Elizabeth has been nothing less than Good Queen Bess.

And yet for some, this is precisely the life category in which the Queen remains most enigmatic, if not somewhat lacking. She is not enormously affectionate and has rarely gone around publicly bestowing hugs and air-kisses on friends or relatives, let alone complete strangers. She wasn't nearly "huggy" enough for Diana, who thought the Queen's approval rating could soar if she, like her, only cuddled a random child now and again.* But the big picture Diana and others like her miss is

---

* It should be noted that Meghan Markle instantly adopted Diana's hugs-and-sympathy approach to a very mixed response in the press. Just three months after her engagement to Prince Harry journalist Jan Moir was already predicting problems. "If only [Meghan] could dial down the full beam of worried sympathy that strobes from her lovely eyes at every opportunity and give it a rest with the endless Lady Bountiful arm-pats, I think people would like her more."

how authentically tenderhearted Elizabeth has always been. As a girl, she was endlessly doling out unsung acts of kindness. Like when she used her wartime-rationed pocket money to buy a poor East End evacuee a proper pair of shoes, or how she voluntarily gave her own ballet slippers to a girl who couldn't afford any (saying they were a spare pair, so the girl wouldn't feel embarrassed), or how she was always the first to write heartfelt letters of sympathy to the mothers of fallen soldiers who previously served at Windsor Castle, making sure to include personalized stories that she remembered each of them by. "For a child of her years," surrounded by such privilege, wrote the King's private secretary Tommy Lascelles, "she has got an astonishing solicitude for other people's comfort; such unselfishness is not a normal characteristic of that family."

Then again, Diana was right. The Queen *does* love differently—treating love less like a visceral feeling than a complex action verb of real contributions made for her family, her country, her Crown and her God. It's a love which has to spread further than most: over more than fifty countries, to be specific. Papua New Guinea, one among many nations where the Queen is head of state, has it about right. There, Elizabeth is better known by the brilliant name "Mama belong big family." But if the Queen has opened her heart to accommodate the masses, she also knows, perhaps more importantly, when to close it for self-protection. Sometimes love means getting out the royal chopping block: loving through lopping off what poses the biggest risks in her life. Elizabeth's heart is anything but squishably "huggy"; Rather it's steady, and self-healing and hugely dependable. Basically it's the stuff royal dreams are made of.

NOBLESSE OBLIGE

OR RULE #17—SOVEREIGN IS
AS SERVANT DOES

There is a motto, which has been borne by many of
my ancestors—a noble motto, "I serve."
—ELIZABETH II

There's nothing like losing thirteen colonies to a bunch of raga-muffin Americans to put things in perspective. In fact, it was probably the best thing that ever happened to the British monarchy. It humbled George III—control freak that he was—and forced him to confront a fast-approaching future where ancient monarchies throughout Europe would be obliterated by modern republics. The real powers of the Crown, even in the late 1700s, had already been chipped away beyond all original reckoning, and George must have wondered where it would all end. How could one ensure the future survival of an inherently privileged institution in this new age of the common man? By looking to the past, as it turned out—specifically, by reaching back to the classical idea of *noblesse oblige*, "nobility obligates," the belief that true greatness is manifested not by looking out for yourself, but by looking out for others. It meant changing from a tyrannical sovereign to the people's servant and, in the process, turning a millennia-old concept of kingship on its head. *Noblesse oblige* transformed George III into the first philanthropist King, causing him to give away more of his own wealth to charity than any previous monarch. And it put his descendants on a trajectory that would both dramatically recast their royal identity and guarantee their long-term survival.

It could be said that for every hospital Queen Victoria opened, every charity she and Albert endorsed, another stone in the defensive wall of public approval was laid. It was not a protection other foreign royals, many of them socially oblivious, spent much time maintaining. So when the tidal wave of anti-monarchial chaos swept Europe in the early twentieth century, the seemingly indestructible thrones of Russia, Germany, Austria-Hungary, Turkey, Italy, Portugal and Greece were all toppled, almost overnight. The de-crowning was so rampant, King Farouk of Egypt predicted that at the current rate of regicide, there would be only five kings left: the king of hearts, diamonds, clubs and spades . . . and the King of England. The House of Windsor was still strongly in the game for good reason. It still held popular power because, as biographer James Pope-Hennessy put it, it was "best defined as the power of doing good"—power which only expanded as time went on. George III's royal household patronized 90 charitable and philanthropic institutions, increasing to 1,200 under Queen Victoria and soaring to around 3,500 under Elizabeth II, a dramatic leap into civic responsibility largely trailblazed by Queen Mary.

*

During World War I Queen Mary earned the affectionate title of "charitable bulldozer" from the press, making sometimes three to four hospital visits each day to console the wounded, while launching a dizzying array of wartime fundraisers and knitting blankets and other comforts like her royal life depended on it. Which in a way, it did. She told as much to a pouty member of the family who, weary of being dragged on yet another hospital visit, once protested, "I'm tired and I hate hospitals." To which Queen Mary replied, "You are a member of the British Royal Family. We are *never* tired, and we all *love* hospitals!"* The memory of

---

* Elizabeth now possesses the same indefatigable spirit. She can attend an endless round of charity events, unveil the same-looking plaque at the same-looking building a thousand times over, watch an innumerable number of children dance or sing with tedious predictability and still retain, like the Queen Mother, "an astonishing gift for being sincerely interested in dull

what becomes of royal selfishness was still painfully fresh. It could easily end, like it did for her Romanov relations, in a cold, dark basement staring into the barrel of a handgun.

Her son Edward's re-embrace of the sovereign's archaic right to be egocentric, consequently, was enormously troubling. Forgetting his own royal motto—*Ich Dien*, "I serve"—Edward childishly shrank into a kingdom of two: himself and his American lover, Wallis Simpson. Thinking of others only cramped his style. Queen Mary begged him to consider how his actions would affect his family, his country, and his empire. But Edward could only reply, "Can't you understand that nothing matters—nothing—except her happiness and mine?" Such was the "motto which, for some years past, had supplanted 'Ich Dien'—and was essentially the underlying principle of his brief reign," said his secretary, Tommy Lascelles. The heady reign of "I don't serve" would last less than a year.

It must have come as a huge relief, then, when Princess Elizabeth showed early signs of un-Edward-like altruism. Her heart for others, for their welfare and comfort, appeared to be innate and, better still, never ostentatious. When one of her earliest and most beloved corgis, "Jane," was accidently run over by a gardener at Windsor, Elizabeth put aside her own sadness to sympathize with the worker, who was seriously shaken by the episode. Putting the blame entirely on herself and her own carelessness, Elizabeth "assured him again and again that it was no fault of his," said her governess. Returning home, she "sat down at once and wrote a most charming note to the gardener" to relieve his conscience further. The same heart would speak, in a few years' time, to her subjects around the world. "It is my resolve that under God I shall not only rule but serve," she told the Australian Parliament in 1954.

We often think the age of royal compassion began and blossomed with Princess Diana, but the Queen got a substantial head start. In 1956 she broke one of the oldest charitable taboos by becoming the first head of state to not only visit a leper colony in Nigeria, but also shake hands

---

people and dull occasions." How does she possibly manage? wondered Charles Robertson, a minister of the Church of Scotland, who had trouble, he admitted, sitting through his own children's school events. The Queen simply replied, "You must set out to enjoy it."

with one of the inhabitants. Since then she has become the patron of a staggering number of charities and public service organizations (totaling 600 when she turned 90), raising billions of pounds for "good causes." They range from the biggies, like cancer research and the British Red Cross, to the tinnies, like the adorable Piobaireachd Society, supporting the heritage of classical bagpipe music (all the Queen is saying is give pipes a chance). The shamelessly republican *Guardian* newspaper has even admitted that "the Queen has done more for charity than any monarch in history."* She receives two hundred to three hundred letters every day, many of them either requests for more charitable patronages or simply personal pleas from her subjects asking for the sovereign's assistance in a variety of problems. If they are a burden on some days, they also are her greatest bulwark: a daily reminder that the Crown is still relevant and relied upon in the modern era. As historian Frank Prochaska sees it, "Barring cataclysm or self-destruction, the monarchy is only likely to be in real danger when the begging letters cease to arrive at Buckingham Palace."

Then again, royal charity is a complex system of cross-pollinating benefits. Flitting from one hospital, fundraiser or community center to the next, it's difficult to tell who has gotten more out of all this bountiful giving: the Windsors or their receiving public? To look closer, however, is to realize that what has saved the British monarchy itself—a devotion to service—has in many ways saved Elizabeth the person too.

*

The Queen touched on the vital importance of service work in 1992, what was self-avowedly the worst year of her life. Reeling from the scandalous collapse of three royal marriages and a devastating fire at Windsor

---

* Even the Queen's clothing choices are an act of service in disguise. They are chosen, above all, with consideration for others in mind. "Her clothes are pretty but never too flamboyant, which might arouse feelings of envy in the crowd," says biographer Ann Morrow. They are consistently brightly colored, so people can easily spot her from a distance. "If I wore beige," Elizabeth has explained, "nobody would know who I am." She also makes a point of carrying transparent umbrellas so people can see her face in the rain and, on international trips, will consciously wear colors that reflect the host country's patriotic hues.

Castle, the Queen's internal compass was recalibrated by continuing to open her heart, not by licking its wounds. Summing up the year in her Christmas broadcast, she said her acts of royal service that year, particularly visiting Group Captain Leonard Cheshire, a disabled World War II hero turned humanitarian, who was bravely enduring a "long drawn-out terminal illness . . . did as much as anything in 1992 to help me put my own worries in perspective." A hundred years before, Queen Victoria made the same connection. The only thing that gradually pulled her out of her comatose grief after Albert's death was the tenacious hook of royal service. It was nothing less than her salvation, thought Lord Clarendon. "The best thing for her," he said, "is the responsibility of her position and the mass of business which she cannot escape from and which during a certain portion of the day compels her to think of something other than the all-embracing sorrow." Without it, Victoria confided to a lady-in-waiting, she would have gladly hopped into the grave with Albert. But "*now* I wish to live and do what I can for my country and those I love," she said.

What is it about giving that makes even the likes of queens (people who seem to have it all) feel more fulfilled? For one, finding happiness by way of a selfless act is a deeply rutted pathway in the human brain. Even toddlers experience the "helpers high"—that warm rush of well-being felt after social acts of kindness or generosity. As studies have shown, toddlers' faces will light up, displaying happier expressions after sharing treats with others in need (in this case, a pretend puppet) than when they originally received the treats themselves. But it's in adulthood when the benefits of giving become most clear. And it goes far beyond warm fuzzies. Acts of altruism are genetically reciprocal. They are the biological equivalent of Newton's third law of motion: for every act of giving there is an equally positive reaction in the giver's body. An occurrence largely due to a powerful anti-inflammatory hormone called oxytocin, a natural stress reliever science has yet to find an equal to. Released whenever we care for others, show compassion or form meaningful social bonds, oxytocin behaves like Bubble Wrap around our most vulnerable innards, especially our heart, protecting them from the damaging pokes of chronic stress and anxiety. When we care for others, "when our compassion circuits are turned on, our angry circuits cannot

be activated. Both circuits can't be on at the same time," says philanthropy expert Jenny Santi. Oxytocin is such a naturally sympathetic
antidote to the human stress response, it's pumped out in our bodies
preemptively at the slightest spike in stress, which biologically prompts
us to turn to others for comfort and relief (which will, in turn, elevate
our protective oxytocin levels). "I find this amazing," says psychologist
Kelly McGonigal. "Your stress response has a built-in mechanism for
stress resilience—and that mechanism is human connection."*

People who knew Diana's anxiety-riddled "other side" were amazed
at her emotional stability when fully engaged with charity work. Habitually drowning in a pool of her own self-pity, helping others became
"her awakening," said Paul Burrell, her butler and confidant. "She truly
felt that her most rewarding time was when she helped the sick and the
dying. She felt 'replenished' by doing it." In Diana's life, it wasn't always
easy to tell where a royal gesture ended and a publicity stunt began, but
her global relief efforts were undeniably driven by the authentic desire
"to feel I am needed." When she got the chance to "support and love"
the world's most vulnerable people, she explained, she felt supported
and loved and a little less vulnerable herself. "They weren't aware just
how much healing they were giving me, and it carried me through." She
later identified the powerful secret of charity work: a mind preoccupied
with others isn't, for that moment, preoccupied with itself. "You don't
think about yourself," she observed, almost with relief, while visiting
land mine victims in Angola.

It was an awakening Diana shared with another princess, Princess
Grace of Monaco (formerly Grace Kelly of Hollywood). Also a royal
outsider accustomed to, as she said, the "easier American attitude toward

---

* Once the helping mechanism is activated, the cascade of benefits can be far-reaching. Studies
have shown that blood pressure, cholesterol, inflammation and BMI numbers dip when people
volunteer regularly. One theory, beyond the effects of oxytocin, is that feeling needed by *others*
might be compelling people to take better care of *themselves*. We are more altruistically motivated than we realize. When researchers compared the efficacy of different handwashing signs
in hospitals, people used far more soap when the notice read "Hand hygiene prevents *patients*
from catching disease" than when the notice read "Hand hygiene prevents *you* from catching
disease."

things," Grace's transition to the rigid protocol of palace life in Monaco was a serious emotional struggle. "During those first years, I lost my identity," she later recalled. What proved pivotal, however, was "when I began service work in Monaco." Among the many altruistic endeavors she threw herself into, Grace rejuvenated the principality's Red Cross, organized the renovation of the dilapidated hospital and made regular home visits to the local elderly. "Then gradually" and almost effortlessly, Grace said, "I joined up with myself again."*

*

Life itself seems to move at a more manageable pace when we give of ourselves. And there are good indications that it can create *more* time, at least from the perspective of the giver. A fascinating set of experiments headed by Yale and Harvard researchers found that when people spent time doing something kind for others—rather than spending time on themselves, like watching TV or self-pampering—their personal sense of time expanded. Writing a five-minute note of encouragement to a sick child, for example, boosted the writer's sense of accomplishment and self-efficacy which, in turn, altered their perceptions of what they could accomplish in a limited amount of time. Helpers felt more time-rich than non-helpers and, as a result, felt they could easily give more of it away. "Giving time gives you time," concluded the researchers. "It sure explains how the typical CEO of any big multinational also happens to sit on a dizzying number of charity boards," says Jenny Santi. Princess Anne certainly makes a good case for the argument. Often dubbed the "hardest working royal," Anne takes on more charitable commitments every year than there are days in the year itself. She fulfilled 640 engagements in 2016 alone. She even found the time to attend a public service event two days after surviving her 1974 kidnapping attempt.

---

* Grace met Diana at the latter's first public event in 1981– a London musical gala—shortly after Diana had become engaged to Prince Charles. Nineteen years old and second-guessing her outfit choice, a tight black dress she herself considered "two sizes too small," Diana poured her wardrobe woes out to a sympathetic Grace who, trying to lighten matters, unknowingly made a poignant prediction. "Don't worry, dear," said Grace, drying Diana's tears in the bathroom, "it'll only get worse."

When a gunman halted her car in London, shot her bodyguard and tried dragging her out of the vehicle at gunpoint, Anne yelled, "Not bloody likely!" (possibly history's pluckiest line) and quickly got back to royal service.

Gaining time through giving it becomes a whole lot more literal when you look long term, at longevity itself. The Queen Mother was convinced that it was "the exhilaration of others" that kept her sprinting past her one-hundredth birthday. Royal service became both her life's purpose and protection rolled into one. "The point of human life and living [is] to give and to create new goodness all the time," she believed. Thinking of others literally got her over the hump on so many occasions. In 2001, aged 100, despite recently breaking her collarbone, she fulfilled all of her previously scheduled engagements, danced a reel after a dinner party in Scotland (so as not to disappoint her guests) and crossed a formidable humpbacked bridge on foot, in order to visit an old and loyal servant who couldn't leave his isolated home in the countryside. All vivid proof of her suspicions that "quite simply, it is the people who keep me up."

Confirmations of her suspicions date back to the 1950s, when scientists first started examining the surprising links between giving and longevity. Studying the life-spans of married women with children, psychologists assumed that the earliest deaths would be among the women with the greatest number of children, due to the increased stress. What they found, however, was the first scientific peek into the long-term benefits of serving others. Life stressors were dramatically reduced—not by having less children but by *helping others*. Women who performed regular volunteer work were less likely to die of a major illness than women who did not volunteer. Near identical evidence has been found in the Nicoya Peninsula of Costa Rica, another global hot spot of longevity, where experts like Dr. Xinia Fernández have been studying the lifestyle patterns of the long-lived Nicoyans. "We noticed that the most highly functioning people over 90 in Nicoya have a few common traits," she told longevity expert Dan Buettner. "One of them is that they feel a strong sense of service to others or care for their family. We see that as soon as they lose this, the switch goes off. They die very quickly if they don't feel needed." A five-year American study of around

1,000 adults in 2013 supported the finding. Despite experiencing major life stressors (which *should* have increased their risk of dying by 30 percent for *each* stressful situation), people who spent time helping others in their lives—family members, neighbors, friends—were spectacularly protected against the risk, showing no occurrence of death from a stress-related cause.

The extraordinary resilience of Philip and Elizabeth, now both in their nineties and both well acquainted with major life stressors, offers ongoing proof of how a heart preoccupied with others can keep on defiantly ticking. Philip's heart, for one, should have puttered out long ago; his temper, his tendency towards grouchiness and abiding hatred of the press have done his cardiovascular system no favors. But with hundreds of charity organizations to personally care for over most of his lifetime (recently totaling 780), Philip has had very limited time to indulge in the irascible behavior that could have killed him many years before.* The job has literally lifted him and the Queen above their own worries and kept them there for over 65 resilient years. Proving that, as Elizabeth once proposed (borrowing a line from the poetry of Adam Lindsay Gordon), when we show "kindness in another's trouble," we enable higher "courage in [our] own."

---

* In all fairness, Philip has always had a very kind and sensitive heart, when he chooses to use it (typically to ameliorate an injustice). As a four-year-old, when staying with family friends in France, he formed a close bond with one of the children, named Ria, who was encased in plaster up to her hips, due to a traumatic fall. He felt outraged when another family visitor came bearing gifts for the other children but callously ignored Ria, reasoning, "you can't play like the others." Philip immediately rushed to his room, collected every toy he possessed and scattered the lot on Ria's bed, exclaiming, "All this is yours!"

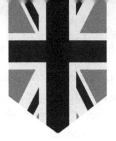

OFF WITH THEIR HEADS

OR RULE #18—AX OUT
YOUR NEED TO BE LIKED

*You don't know that you are saying these things to a princess,
and that if I chose I could wave my hand and order you to execution.
I only spare you because I am a princess, and you are a poor, stupid,
unkind, vulgar old thing, and don't know any better.*

—Frances Hodgson Burnett, *A Little Princess*

O nce upon a more chivalrous time, the Queens and Kings of England were afforded the rather handy accessory of a "Champion" fighter—someone to literally throw down the gauntlet and lance any ruffian who slandered or spoke ill of the monarch's right to rule. Galloping into Westminster Hall in full armor, the Champion would herald the Arthurian equivalent of *them's fightin' words!* ("If any person, of whatever degree soever, high or low, shall deny or gainsay our Sovereign . . . here is her Champion, who saith that he lieth, and is a false traitor, being ready in person to combat with him, and in this quarrel will adventure his life against him . . ."), allowing the Queen to yawn in the dependable certainty that her honor would be upheld, without lifting a bejeweled finger. At least that was the original theory. By 1830, however, William IV—strapped for cash—thought he could fight his own battles more economically, so the office of Champion went the way of other courtly nonessentials (like the Royal Falconer and, alas, the Royal Herb Strewer*). The titles still exist, but only ceremonially. Until recently, the Queen's hereditary "Champion" was a chartered accountant from Lincolnshire. Much good that will do.

No, in facing those who prove less than loyal, Elizabeth has needed to become her own champion, defending herself against all attacks, especially those that seek to ruffle the inner peace of her personal kingdom. But whereas her predecessors dealt with undesirables at the end of an ax, Elizabeth has found other ways to mete out royal justice, surprisingly just as effectively. M'lords and ladies, I give you Her Majesty's tough love.

＊

Every modern royal, at some point, will harbor secret fantasies for returning to the swift delights of the rack and the chopping block. Especially on the days when, say, a once trusted staff member writes a best-selling tell-all, betraying years of royal confidence for a quick buck, or when a scuzzy reporter decimates your reputation with a cruel headline based on nothing but gossip and hearsay. For Princess Anne—never one to mince words—a good old Norman shake-up would serve admirably on such occasions. "I am tempted to suggest the reintroduction of the Norman law," she says, "where a slanderer not only had to pay damages but was also liable to stand in the marketplace of the nearest town, hold his nose between two fingers and confess himself to be a liar." Rather mild, all things considered, especially when you take into account the current Windsor recompense for those who have seriously displeased the Crown.

Terrifyingly referred to as the "freeze out" by biographer Elizabeth Longford, it's the silent treatment on royal steroids, when offenders don't just stop receiving an annual Christmas card from the Palace, they become "non-persons" as far as the Windsor's are concerned,

---

* Once charged with the lovely—if somewhat vapid—regal purpose of scattering aromatic herbs and flowers during royal processions, the position of Royal Herb Strewer went to Anne Fellowes in 1821. The Fellowes family has *loosely* laid claim to the title ever since—making the current Royal Herb Strewer one Jessica Fellowes, niece of the selfsame Julian Fellowes, creator of *Downton Abbey*. It's a small English world after all.

experiencing a sharp severance of whatever contact and communication they might have previously enjoyed. Biographer Ingrid Seward calls it "the equivalent of being sent to the Tower in another age." It doesn't happen often, but once the icy curtain has fallen, the freeze out is usually permanent.

Enter the hapless Marion Crawford, once sitting pretty as Elizabeth and Margaret's retired governess, granted unrestricted access to the royal family and a grace-and-favor house at Kensington Palace. That is, until she listened to her mercenary husband who convinced her that the plaudits and purse strings of a curious public were more worth pursuing. Soon penning *The Little Princesses*, a life-with-the-Windsors memoir, it was the first book of its kind, a staff reveal-all shattering sixteen years of implicit royal confidence for the seduction of quick cash. It would be Crawfie's worst mistake. Now utterly unable to be trusted by the people who cherished her most, she experienced the full force of the royal freeze out. She never saw the Windsors again, retreated to Scotland where she wobbled towards a nervous breakdown and eventually lost the public's trust as well, when it was later discovered that her continuing "in person" coverage of royal events for magazines were presumptive lies, written six weeks in advanced. Her death in 1988 saw no flowers sent from the royal family she had betrayed in such a way that made renewal of the relationship impossible. To this day, "doing a Crawfie" is Palace euphemism for any shortsighted act of betrayal that permanently sells out the Queen's trust.

Unsurprisingly, Elizabeth has kept the number of her friends and confidants down to a safe minimum. Past courtiers like Eileen Parker estimated that the number of people "intimate enough to address" the Queen by her first name adds up to only about a dozen. Many of them are simply "nice dull people," as the Queen Mother liked to say, but "valuable" as "gold" for that very reason. Elizabeth does not want or need any more. "The Crown" might have "a lonely splendour," as Tennyson poetically wrote, but there is undeniable safety in the splendor of the few.*

---

* Prince Philip would prove the wisdom "you are the company you keep." During the 1950s he became chummy with a group of wealthy men with too much time and libido on their hands. Collectively known as the Thursday Club, they met once a week for lunch and

The Queen can be incredibly friendly, but those who wish to ingratiate themselves as her new BFF quickly realize the insurmountable difference between royal friendliness and friendship. Elizabeth doesn't like to confuse the two, becoming an expert at keeping her distance in the politest way possible. She is Britain's "slightly mysterious Department of Friendliness," says Andrew Marr. One of her most effective strategies lies simply in the way she shakes people's hands. Those who clasp on to the royal glove too long will find their own hand promptly returned to them. Actress Claire Foy, who played Elizabeth in *The Crown*, says "she's the inventor of the 'shove back.' She really gives you your hand back after you've met her."

But the Queen can strategically *keep her distance* in her own family, as well, when required—something which Prince Philip has benefited from most. He might be her "strength and stay" of over seventy years, but he has also been irritating, testy, critical, grumbly, cruel and isn't shy of calling the Queen "a bloody fool" when his dander is up. During such moments, Elizabeth makes every effort to remove "herself from the blistering line of fire," says biographer Carolly Erickson. "I'm simply not going to appear," the Queen would say, "until Philip is in a better temper." Elizabeth believes that emotions are catching, like the common cold. In the same way that, as she puts it, "kindness, sympathy, resolution and courteous behavior are infectious," so too is anger, frustration and hostility. She's right. Psychologists call it "emotional contagion"—the way negativity can unwittingly spread from one individual to another. A rotten mood can rub off within seconds, making distance the safest way to de-escalate the conflict and avoid getting splattered with negativity yourself. Queen Mary was a master in spousal-distancing. Whenever her husband, George V, would reduce a family dinner to a tirade of rages and rude remarks, Queen Mary would simply rise from the table and lead her children silently out of the room.

Practicing the same herself, Elizabeth has undoubtedly preserved what is now the longest-enduring marriage in British royal history. She

---

licentious humor at a restaurant in Soho. It turned out to be a den of scandal, of indiscreet name-droppers and of chronically unfaithful husbands. Philip was tainted by association, sparking rumors of his own infidelities that have haunted him ever since.

might throw in the odd "Oh, do shut up, Philip" when he is especially exasperating but, by and large, Philip is the first to admit that if "tolerance is the one essential ingredient" in a marriage, then "you can take it from me that the Queen has the quality of tolerance in abundance." It's been the same for her adult children and her perpetually childish sister, Margaret. The Queen preserved their sisterly bond by simply refusing to stoop to Margaret's emotional histrionics. Like the time Margaret telephoned a friend, interrupting his house party with the frantic report that, being near suicide, if he didn't come over immediately, she would soon be throwing herself out the window. The concerned friend immediately rang the Queen, who could be heard audibly rolling her eyes on the other line. "Carry on with your house party," said the Queen coolly. "Her bedroom is on the ground floor." Stoics like Elizabeth will often treat misbehaving relations "as if they were small children throwing a tantrum," says Donald Robertson, a cognitive behavioral psychotherapist. It makes little sense to get angry at such immature outbursts. Call it tolerance or simply common sense, the long-term results have been self-evident. The more he witnessed the royal drama unfold, the more Louis Mountbatten believed that keeping her family together and coping with their self-inflicted messes was the Queen's greatest personal achievement. More so when you consider, as Mountbatten told his confidant John Barratt, that while "most people can hide their family difficulties . . . hers are always the focus of public attention." Yet for the Queen, it's always been the bigger picture, not the isolated tiffs with her children, grandchildren, husband or sister, that have most concerned her. She still believes, as her mother did before her, that "a united family is the strongest thing in the world."* Especially when a family is forced to unite against an unpredictable ex-King.

---

* One of the Queen's unspoken rules is to never talk badly about any member of her family to outsiders, rather only support them, when she can. Diana might have made her life unimaginably difficult in the 1990s, but the Queen quickly jumped to her defense when, during a press conference at the Palace, an editor of the *News of the World* inquired that if Diana didn't want paparazzi following her, couldn't she send a servant to run her errands for her? "That's the most pompous thing I have ever heard," responded the Queen, famously earning a round of applause from the other editors in the room.

※

In the 1930s Edward VIII's refusal to step down from the office of kingship quietly—foolishly flirting with the Nazi idea to install him as a puppet king if Germany won the war—meant he incurred a "freeze out" of monumental proportions. Those left to pick up the pieces of his abdication crisis closed ranks, including the Palace staff, who were more than happy to raise the drawbridges behind their former boss. "One can only wonder what a mess we might have had if Edward stayed on," said one member of the household after Edward's departure. "Wonder on your own time!" retorted Tommy Lascelles. "And don't mention him again." The Duke of Windsor in name only now, Edward was barred from his brother's and niece's coronation and was only mildly tolerated at Queen Mary's funeral, but was explicitly *not* invited to dine at Windsor Castle afterward. The freeze out made Edward furious. Writing to Wallis, he snarked, "What a smug stinking lot my relations are, and you've never seen such a seedy worn out bunch of old hags most of them have become." Just one of the many spiteful remarks he would blast about the new Elizabethan court. Luckily, the Queen doesn't mind being disliked.

She knows she can't please everyone and doesn't attempt to try. It's a sincerity, a bravery to be oneself, that has long been a hallmark of the English upper classes. As the cultural historian Sarah Lyall explains, unlike the country's social-climbing middle classes, "true aristocrats are perhaps the only people in Britain secure enough not to care how others view [them]. . . . British aristocrats feel no need to impress people." Nor will they say or do things to get others to like them more. Elizabeth will laugh or smile only when she is genuinely amused. There is no trace of "the political perma-smile" about her, says reporter Kevin Sullivan, impressed by the Queen's unaffected "habit of smiling only when she finds something funny." It's the great irony of the role she inhabits, itself full of showy pomp and a fair bit of pretense. Yet "at the heart of Britain's performing monarchy," explains the historian Robert Lacey, "is a serious, matter-of-fact woman who is an obstinate nonperformer."*

---

* Of course, no one pulled off this royal insouciance better than Princess Margaret. She was *always* her sassy self. Consider the dinner party when Lord Carnarvon offered her a glass of

It's a deep integrity to self that extends to the Queen's speeches as well. Her fakeness radar is so sensitive, when Martin Charteris once presented her with a draft for a speech that innocuously began "I am very glad to be back in Birmingham," she honed in on the "very" and crossed it out, explaining that it was no slight on Birmingham itself, she just couldn't bear what seemed to her like an insincere exaggeration. Moreover, she doesn't feign interest in modern art or read trendy books that other people say she should like. If she reads for pleasure at all, it's rumored to be detective stories or lowbrow tales about horses. And most importantly, she will never confuse those who genuinely annoy her with mock signals of friendliness. One way or another, you will always know where you stand with the Queen. The British actress Miriam Margolyes (known both for her role as Professor Sprout in the *Harry Potter* films and for her brusque, unmannerly outbursts) recently attended a Palace function and, getting loquaciously carried away as usual, rudely interrupted the Queen as she was talking to another guest. "Be quiet," said the Queen bluntly, prioritizing her own personal standards over being palsy-walsy with Professor Sprout.

*

"The trouble with behaving like everyone else is that you get treated like everyone else," Martin Charteris once quipped. "The Queen has succeeded because she has never done that." Though it could be said that other royals, like Sarah Ferguson, failed so miserably for the same reason, only reversed. Sarah was excruciatingly uncomfortable with being disliked. A bit of bad press in the tabloids "kidnapped my sleep and composure for days on end," she recalls. She needed *every-one's* approval to feel whole, even complete strangers. When a baggage

---

exquisitely rare Madeira from 1836. Holding his breath for her reaction, Margaret took one sip and promptly proclaimed it "Exactly like petrol." Or the time Elizabeth Taylor made a surprise debut at a small gathering of the princess's friends at Kensington Palace. Expecting the usual Hollywood treatment, Taylor stood waiting in the doorway for an awkward amount of time. One friend attempted to rouse Margaret to the situation. "Oh Ma'am, Elizabeth Taylor has just arrived!" Margaret simply let out a sigh, saying, "Oh, well I suppose somebody had better offer her a drink!"

handler at the airport once overheard her express mild exhaustion after a long trip overseas, he rather loudly mumbled, "You don't know what work is." Sarah couldn't bear the slight. "Oh please don't say that," she pleaded with the man. "You don't realise that I do have to work hard. Please don't believe what you read in the newspapers." The fact that she had, just moments ago, been proud of her hard work "wasn't enough," said Sarah. "No, I couldn't be satisfied until this stranger became my friend." Entering the royal family on a high wave of public approval ("Great-Fun Fergie" was going to permanently liven up the Palace, the press predicted), she couldn't cope when the inevitable troughs came. Overly reliant on other people's opinions and approval, she internalized the worst the press could throw at her: "[I] completely believed every single thing they wrote. I believed I was the worthless person they were talking about."*

Oliver Cromwell, for all his anti-monarchial madness, had the right idea. He might have executed Charles I and popularly installed himself as Lord Protector of England, but he wasn't going to let the adulation go to his head. Riding through the cheering streets of London in 1650, Cromwell told his companions that, yes, he was very pleased by the enormous show of support, but he also knew that the same crowds would likely gather, just as uproariously, to see him hanged. Today, no one can confirm the dizzying swings of public approval better than Prince Charles. It's hard to believe that, prior to Diana, Charles was once voted the most likable member of the royal family. Seventy percent of the county once thought so. But by 1993 his approval rating had

---

* Years later, Sarah made a discovery that would behoove every future royal to remember. Touring the offices of a British newspaper, Sarah met the writer responsible for, at one time, churning out hurtful zingers, like the infamous "Duchess of Pork" headline. Doubtless expecting a suave villain with a curly moustache, Sarah was shocked as a fat, balding, rather jovial fellow introduced himself. "You caused me great distress, you know," Sarah told him. "Oh dear, I didn't mean to," said the man, explaining that, from his end, the headline was generated simply because *Pork* rhymed with *York*. "He was paid to be clever, end of story," concluded Sarah. "Where I once took his every pun so personal, he'd invested no more emotion in them than he would in his tie clasp . . . It occurred to me that we survive our critics by knowing that their agendas, at heart, may have little to do with us."

plummeted to an almost invisible 4 percent. A number which has gradually risen again, incidentally, as Charles has become more comfortable in his own skin and less worried about what other people think of the projects and causes dear to his heart. The thousands of people who have benefited from these projects must be grateful that Charles didn't give up, basing his inner worth on his outward popularity. As Ichiro Kishimi and Fumitake Koga explain in their best-selling *The Courage to Be Disliked*, there is a certain "freedom in being disliked by other people," as "it is proof that you are exercising your freedom and living in freedom, and a sign that you are living in accordance with your own principles."

For eight years Australian palliative caregiver Bronnie Ware listened to the parting words of the dying, noting the surprising commonalities of their deepest regrets. Repeated time and again, the number one regret of the dying wasn't a lack of fame or constant approval, but a lack of personal courage to be themselves. That is "I wish I'd had the courage to live a life true to myself, not the life others expected of me." Prince Philip has extended practically the same advice, albeit with his usual pragmatic spunk. "The idea that you don't do anything on the off-chance you might be criticized" is futile, he says. "You'd end up living like a cabbage and it's pointless." In short, be yourself and be willing to be disliked, even if you're the Queen. An observer at a West End performance that Elizabeth and the Queen Mother were attending once overheard a slight argument in the royal box. "Who do you think you are?" asked the elder in a decorous whisper. Elizabeth confidently whispered back, "The Queen, mummy, the Queen."

SOME ONE ELSE

OR RULE #19—DEFEND THE FAITH
WHICH DEFENDS YOU

More things are wrought by prayer than this world dreams of.
—ALFRED TENNYSON, *IDYLLS OF THE KING*

To casually reach for a one-pound coin in modern Britain is to tender an idea older than coinage itself. Engraved on the coin's surface, after the Queen's name, are the almost code-like letters D-G-REG. The abbreviated rendering of *Dei Gratia Regina,* "by the grace of God," is a stunning acknowledgment, especially in a secular age, that the monarch's power and position doesn't derive from the government or the consent of the people, but directly from God, the ultimate Sovereign.* The idea has seen its historical hiccups, to be sure. Abusing the "divine right of kings" ended disastrously for Charles I and embarrassingly for King Canute, who couldn't quite get the ocean's tidal currents to obey his godlike command. But it has also been a transcending power for good, creating historic stability through the reassuring belief that, as Shakespeare would say, "this blessed plot, this earth, this realm, this England" is held together by more than the

---

* The coin's full inscription reads: ELIZABETH II D-G-REG-F-D, with the final "F-D" meaning *Fidei Defensor,* "Defender of the Faith." First stamped on British coins in 1714, the notation was removed on a two-shilling piece in 1849, causing such public outrage toward the so-called "Godless Florin," the coin had to be promptly reissued with its traditional message.

sum of its political parts. Unlike the earthbound whims of elected politicians, "people see the monarchy" differently, says biographer Elizabeth Longford, as something which "has not been entirely fabricated by themselves, man-made . . . making it seem to reach out into a world beyond." England lasted little more than one shaky decade as a republic in the mid-seventeenth century—incidentally, a time when its highest powers reached no higher than fallible men. The country has always needed something bigger to construct its democratic scaffold upon. And the monarchy, perhaps, has needed it most of all. When your face is on every coin, stamp and banknote in the land, it's crucial to know that Some One Else is higher still.

"Some One Else" was George VI's insightful expression, referencing a numinous moment during his coronation of 1937. As the Archbishop readied the King for the most holy rite of the ceremony—the anointing with oil—George said he experienced a powerful awareness that, besides the Archbishop, "Some One Else was with him" under the royal canopy. Observes felt it too: "It seemed that these two men were alone with God, performing an act greater than they knew, more solemn than any person present could hope to understand." Elizabeth herself would go under the canopy just two decades later. "The Queen's Hallowing," as it was called—the moment she exchanged her exquisite robes for a simple white dress, when she was uniquely blessed by the Archbishop—was, in Elizabeth's mind, the moment she truly passed into Queenship. The spiritual blessing made her Queen, not the act of putting on a crown or saying a few lofty oaths. The anointing was considered so sacred at the time, the live television cameras around Westminster Abbey—the first at any British coronation—deferentially panned away. Filming the rite felt like prying into a deeply personal pact between God and the Queen. Even today, watching the black-and-white 1953 coronation film, it's hard not to be moved. At the time, its spiritual impacts were palpably felt around the country. Post-coronation Britain witnessed its greatest faith revival since the mid-nineteenth century, with dramatic increases in church membership, baptisms, communions, Sunday school enrollment and religious marriages. It was an almost mystical time when vast numbers of Britons still truly believed, like Princess Margaret, that the Queen was "God's representative in this realm." Times have certainly changed. But while equally vast numbers of her subjects have, today, abandoned their spiritual heritage on an unprecedented scale, the Queen has resolutely held on as firm as ever.

＊

Her Christian faith "is the absolute mainspring of her life," says Bishop Michael Mann, the former Dean of Windsor. "The Queen is a person of very deep faith." She attends church every Sunday, without fail, and ends every day on her knees, beside her bed, in prayer. As a girl, mornings for Elizabeth began in her mother's bedroom, reading a chapter of the Bible together, swathing her in spiritual truths she has relied on ever since. "While she may guard her feelings in other ways," says Mark Greene, who has written about the Queen's enduring faith, "about Jesus she has been remarkably, one might say, uncharacteristically open about what she believes." He is her self-avowed "inspiration," her "role model" and her "anchor." People who would like to see a little more spiritual agnosticism from the Queen, especially in her Christmas broadcasts, forget that, among her many historic titles is "Defender of the Faith." Pope Leo X conferred the title on Henry VIII in 1521, and it has since been born by each successive monarch. For Elizabeth, defending the faith means reminding people, particularly in an age where spiritual ambivalence has led to historically high levels of personal emptiness, not to, as she says, "carelessly throw away ageless ideals" that have supported the human condition for innumerable generations. "I know just how much I rely on my faith to guide me through the good times and the bad," she told her subjects in 2002. "I know that the only way to live my life is to try to do what is right, to take the long view, to give of my best in all that the day brings and to put my trust in God."

The Queen has a strong "external locus of control," as psychologists call it—the comfort in knowing that Some One Else is ultimately in charge. In the words of the Duchess of York, the Queen might be driving the car of monarchy, but she also knows she is "not what makes the engine go." It was Elizabeth's idea, in fact, to share with her father a simple poem that would famously encapsulate the idea. Searching for the right words for his 1939 Christmas broadcast, in the early doubt-ridden days of World War II, George VI was handed a few memorable lines by Princess Elizabeth, then age thirteen, who thought they might help:

> And I said to the man who stood at the gate of the year: "Give me a light that I may tread safely into the unknown." And he replied: "Go out into the darkness and put your hand into the Hand of God. That shall be to you better than light and safer than a known way."

Elizabeth was right. The spiritual reminder brought comfort to millions, rousing their courage through the conviction that they weren't alone in the fight. Despair, nihilism, and crippling fears are not viable options when you believe, like the Queen does, that the "Prince of Peace" has your back. For George Carey, the former Archbishop of Canterbury, faith is the deepest foundation stone of Elizabeth's iconic stamina: "She's got a capacity because of her faith to take anything the world throws at her. Her faith comes from a theology of life that everything is ordered." The same pattern surfaced time and again in Dan Buettner's investigation of the longest-lived individuals around the world. Relinquishing worries to a higher power was a universal pathway to emotional and physical resilience. "Healthy centenarians everywhere have faith," he concluded, identifying belief as "a great stress reducer for these people" at the very least. "The fact that God is in control of their lives relieves any economic, spiritual, or well-being anxiety they might otherwise have. They go through life with the peaceful certitude that someone is looking out for them."*

---

* In 2009 one of the most prestigious scientific journals, *Psychological Bulletin*, published data confirming that religious devotion does indeed affect longevity. Reviewing hundreds of studies that tracked test subjects over time, researchers found that nonreligious individuals expired sooner than religiously active people. Healthier lifestyle choices among people of faith are the usual explanation, but it could be deeper than that. A Duke University study demonstrated that regular churchgoers had lower markers of interleukin-6 in their blood, a protein which, when elevated, may indicate a weakened immune system. And a Stanford University study of over 100 women with metastatic breast cancer found that those with more religious expression in their lives had higher immune-boosting white blood cell counts.

The Queen likewise deals with tragedies by tapping into the calmer waters of her faith—a fact the secular press shamefully ignored in 1997. The day after Diana died, Elizabeth was roundly attacked for attending Sunday church service, as usual, with her grandsons William and Harry. The act was instantly sneered at by journalists who couldn't fathom the idea that comfort could exist in anything other than laying cellophane-wrapped flowers outside the gates of Kensington Palace. Yet William and Harry both wanted a more secure scaffold for their grief. They wanted to go to church "to talk to Mummy," as William told his grandmother. People who have completely disassociated themselves from religious tradition forget, says biographer Gyles Brandreth, that "there is comfort to be had from familiar hymns and prayers. There is solace to be found in form and custom long-established."

Unsurprisingly, traditional Christianity has always been the Queen's spiritual bread and butter. She prefers the ancient, quiet liturgy of the Anglican Church to more flamboyant evangelical styles. Her go-to is still the 1662 version of the Book of Common Prayer and the King James translation of the Bible. Yet she has never been dogmatic about the finer mysteries of the Christian faith (she was the first British monarch to meet a Catholic pope since the Reformation). Nor does she delight, like Philip does, in dissecting every theological argument down to its sinewy nubs. As it was with the Queen Mother, Elizabeth's faith is both "traditional and uncomplicated," says biographer William Shawcross. She believes, as she hinted in 2000, that "the Christian message" can be summed up in eight lines or less:*

> Go forth into the world in peace,
> Be of good courage,
> Hold fast that which is good,

---

* Perhaps explaining the Queen's antipathy for long sermons. A snappy, seven-minute homily is her ideal, "believing that if a preacher could not make his point in this time he never would," says biographer Ingrid Seward. Elizabeth and Philip both greatly appreciated Michael Mann, the Dean of Windsor from 1976 to 1989, for this reason. He kept his sermons mercifully short. As Philip has pithily put it, "the mind and soul cannot absorb what the buttock cannot bear."

Render to no man evil for evil,
Strengthen the faint hearted,
Support the weak,
Help the afflicted,
Honour all men.

Religion, as its root implies, "binds" us to these self-aligning truths, to deeper realities science, technology and materialism can never articulate or answer for. Prince Philip, who has restlessly toyed with every alternative philosophy on the planet, has, time and again, reached the same conclusion. "Religious conviction," he says, "is the strongest and probably the only factor in sustaining the dignity and integrity of the individual." Princess Diana's life sadly proved the point. She spread her spiritual safety blanket so thin with ambiguous beliefs, it was practically invisible to both herself and others. "The long caravan of advisers, astrologers, clairvoyants, counsellors, gurus, homeopaths, hypnotherapists, 'lifestyle managers', mystics, New Age therapists, personal trainers, psychotherapists, sleep therapists, soothsayers and tarot card readers whom she allowed into her life," says journalist Jeremy Paxman, only "disclosed her own inner vulnerability." Making the public's hyper-confused reaction to her death perhaps inevitable. Not knowing what she truly believed in life, it was difficult for others to find the slightest consolation in her passing. It shows "what happens when all beliefs have parity of esteem," continues Paxman. "Those who put their trust in princes and princesses want them to put their own trust in something more than a passing snake-oil salesman."

*

It is largely for her country, therefore, that the Queen recharges every day through the stabilizing act of prayer. Starting in childhood, morning and evening prayers—the latter done with hands clasped, by her bedside—have been "as much a part of [her] daily life as brushing [her] hair and getting dressed," says biographer Ingrid Seward. Perhaps in the most uniquely symbolic way possible, prayer is the one outlet through which the Queen can feel gloriously lesser-than, when she can cast her heavy crown with all its worries and aspirations at the foot of a higher Throne.

"For Christians, as for all people of faith, reflection, mediation and prayer helps us to renew ourselves in God's love," says Elizabeth. Anyone who has made prayer a part of their daily routine can relate to its unmatchable powers to simultaneously relax and reinnervate—the best way to start the day with promise, as the Queen does, and end it with peace. No one can be royal at heart without it, insists Prince Alexi Lubomirski. Writing to his children on prayer's life-changing importance, he counsels, "Whether in a church, a field, on a mountaintop, walking to school or in your bedroom, pray. Have conversations with God."

One day when the Queen herself passes away, sadness will engulf the nation, to be sure, but, unlike with Diana's passing, mass misery and angry bewilderment almost certainly will not. This is not because Elizabeth has been any less loved—her Diamond Jubilee in 2012 turned out more crowds than William and Kate's wedding, after all—but because her subjects know, deep down, that she loved and was loved by Some One more eternal than England itself. This truth will ease her passing as it has unquestionably eased her life. The Queen enjoys a transcendent hope that was once shared by the majority of her subjects: the assurance, as historian Peter Ackroyd records, that "life was only the beginning, not the end, of existence." There will always be those who trivialize such a conviction, but it's difficult to ignore the comfort and profound courage it has instilled in Elizabeth's life.* You can see it every time she does an exposed walkabout in a crowd or rides in an open carriage (when, at any moment, a crazed gunman could open fire). Believing she is bound for another world has, ironically, grounded her more in this one. Death for the Queen, in the words of one of her kingly predecessors, will be the simple exchange of a corruptible crown for an incorruptible one. The result: she can be fully present and at peace, whatever the day might bring. As one of her close friends has put it, "she has her luggage packed and is ready to go."

---

* Even the highly intelligent German philosopher Nietzsche, who hastily announced "God is dead" in the nineteenth century, recognized that people still need the hope of eternity as an antidote against nihilism. The best he could come up with, barring God, was the "eternal recurrence" theory—a rather depressing riff on reincarnation, where the universe and everything in it (including yourself) relives its existence, in the same exact way, an infinite number of times.

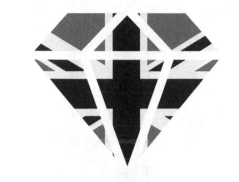

Age Like
a Queen

May heaven, great monarch,
still augment your bliss,
With length of days,
and every day like this!

—JOHN DRYDEN

Be willing to be old.

—GEORGE MACDONALD

On September 23, 1896, Queen Victoria broke the longevity record. Her journal entry that day proudly marks the occasion. She had officially beaten George III's hitherto longest reign by one day, edging out his distinction of 59 years and 96 days. She had done it. She had ostensibly fulfilled the final and most elusive of all hopes contained in the English national anthem: "Long to reign over us." But she got there practically collapsing at the milestone. At 78, Victoria was morbidly obese and hardly able to walk. Her Diamond Jubilee, which should have celebrated her persistent vitality, was reduced to a drive-through event. Unable to mount the 24 steps into St. Paul's Cathedral, Victoria pulled up alongside the building and waited as the congregation came out to her, commemorating her 60 years on the throne, as it were, stuck inside her carriage. That alone was exhausting enough. And Victoria, frail and full of rheumatic pain, limited all jubilee celebrations to that single day.

The next Diamond Jubilee Britain celebrated—only the second in its history—would be astonishingly different. Elizabeth, aged 86, spent a jam-packed year marking the occasion, culminating in a four-day frenzy of events in June of 2012, including a floating pageant on the River Thames, during which Elizabeth stood for nearly four hours on an unusually cold, rainy day waving to her subjects (with nary a lean against the purpose-built "throne" provided for her). A couple of days later, though it hardly bears mentioning, she easily climbed the steps of St. Paul's that once proved insurmountable to Victoria.

It illustrates an important distinction: the difference between longevity as a pure numerical feat, due to little more than genetics, and longevity as a thriving, energetic result of smart personal decisions. As Elizabeth likes to say, quoting Groucho Marx, "Anyone can get old—all you have to do is to live long enough." But to age gracefully is a different matter entirely. To age with your mind and body still supple and sharp, your zest for life still strong, takes more than a handful of good Hanoverian genes.* You might say it takes a bit of *la reyne le veult,* an age-old Norman expression meaning "the Queen wills it." It's still used whenever the Queen gives her consent to acts of Parliament and rather nicely encapsulates her attitude towards aging well itself. That is, it rarely happens without one's consent. Elizabeth's comfortable acceptance of the passing years might seem effortless, her survival magical even, but beneath the surface is a determined, defiant, fabulous willingness to make her last royal act the most happy and glorious yet.

---

* Roughly 75 percent more. That's how much people's life-spans are believed to be determined by lifestyle habits and environmental factors. Only about 25 percent is dictated by genes, according to a seminal study of Danish twins who, while sharing nearly identical genetic profiles, were raised in different environments.

RADIANCE

OR RULE #20—MORE PERMANENCE, LESS PLASTIC SURGERY

To be stable in so public a position is not enough;
one must look stable as well.
—JAMES POPE-HENNESSY

I did not feel my best, but I did not let it show. I kept clutching
my red Hermès bag, which matched my red hat and red jacket.
Chic colour co-ordination counts, even in an emergency.
—PRINCESS MICHAEL OF KENT, ON SURVIVING AN EMERGENCY HELICOPTER LANDING

Up until fairly recently, the worst royal portrait the Queen had to put up with was Pietro Annigoni's 1969 painting, which looks desolate, unfinished and slightly creepy. In it, a military-garbed Elizabeth seems to be channeling the Elf Queen from *The Lord of the Rings* film, ready to toss back her crimson robe to declare, "In place of a Dark Lord you would have a Queen!" That all changed in 2001 when artist Lucian Freud, the 79-year-old grandson of Sigmund Freud (red flags right there), unveiled *Her Majesty the Queen*, after making the art world wait nearly a year for his promised masterpiece. What they got was a heavily blotched, awkwardly small canvas smeared with the depiction of what looks like, to be frank, an ugly drag queen with a five-o'clock shadow. The nation was beside itself with indignation.

"It makes her look like one of the royal corgis who has suffered a stroke," said Robert Simon, editor of the *British Art Journal.* "Freud should be locked in the Tower for this," raged photographer Arthur Edwards. To art critic Adrian Searle, someone who tried to keep an open mind, the Queen's painted grimace was reminiscent of the "'before' half of a before-and-after testimonial for constipation tablets." The *Sun* pronounced it "a travesty." The painting's unveiling was, in short, oddly destabilizing. That an unflattering portrait, barely the size of a sheet of paper, should wildly offend an entire nation, however, isn't odd when you consider its deeper significance. The Queen's "look" has long been entwined with the symbolic identity of her people. Her body still represents "the body politic" of Britain itself.* Her outward radiance is reflective of the country's inner spirit. What Freud's scowling old woman said about Britain wasn't just insulting, it was patently untrue. Attempting to be clever and "realistic," it distorted the true reality of a life that has aged remarkably well. The *Daily Telegraph* said it best, conceding that the Queen might "no longer [be] the heart-breakingly beautiful woman she was [once]," but like the best of historic Britain, she is still "easy on the eye."

Elizabeth has always looked younger than her numerical age suggests. A softening began early when, well into young adulthood, she dressed either similarly or exactly like Margaret, younger by four years, allowing her sibling, it was said, "to catch up." But nothing has quite softened Elizabeth's appearance over the decades like her famously youthful skin. Called many splendid things—"porcelain," "sparkling" and the usual favorite, "radiant,"—there hasn't been a biography of the Queen written that hasn't, in some way, paid homage to her royal epidermis. The first

---

* The medieval doctrine that the monarch had a "body politic" in addition to his or her natural body proved of vital importance to Britain's female rulers. Elizabeth I, in particular, could never have secured her rule without it. It essentially guaranteed she would be respected as a man, by other men, at a time when women were flagrantly disregarded as the inferior sex. Since the Queen uniquely embodied the identity of a Crown and country which transcended gender—"the body politic"—her pesky womanhood was conveniently overlooked in all matters of state. As Elizabeth I reminded her all-male assembly of lords in 1558, "I am but one body naturally considered, though by [God's] permission a body politic to govern."

time Martin Charteris met Elizabeth, he "was immediately struck by her bright blue eyes and her wonderful complexion." The photographer Cecil Beaton was dazzled by her "sugar pink" cheeks. Ditto the Baron of Brabourne who, upon seeing the Queen in the flesh, remarked to Philip, "I never realized what lovely skin she has." To which Philip inappropriately replied (big surprise), "She's like that all over." For many, this is exactly where Freud's painting fell so blatantly short. As biographer Sally Bedell Smith observes, Freud's blotchy orange brushstrokes failed to capture the "luminous skin" the Queen still possesses in old age, largely due, as Smith notes, to her "healthy living, and an unfussy beauty regimen."

"The Queen's creamy and supple complexion," said royal writer Ann Morrow, "is an example to any woman who likes to think that expensive cosmetics are the secret of a good skin." For years, Elizabeth used a variety of reasonably priced Cyclax products on her face, including their Milk of Roses moisturizer. She also believes less is definitely more when it comes to makeup. A quick puff of powder and a coat of bright lipstick (like the "Balmoral" shade she commissioned in 1952 to match her coronation robes) has been her only iconic embellishments. All of which she applies herself—only recruiting the assistance of a professional makeup artist one day out of the entire year, for her annual Christmas broadcast. Her dressing table has never been the secret of her youthful radiance.* Her wardrobe is a different story.

※

---

* With the possible exception of how the Queen washes her face. It's not entirely clear, but Elizabeth may follow the Queen Mother's strictures on face washing. Namely, don't do it. Not with soap, at least. Explaining the Queen Mother's glorious complexion to an observer, George VI once remarked, "Do you know she has never washed her face in her life? I did not believe it before I was married but I know it's so. She puts some grease stuff on at night & it rubs off on the pillow by morning & that is all she ever does." The Queen later corrected him, saying she *did* use a cold cream in place of soap, but she washed it off with plenty of cool water. Interestingly, another royal known for her flawless skin, Princess Grace of Monaco, said the same. Her image might have once been used in ads for Lux soap—to get that "movie star complexion"—but she confided the real secret to a journalist years later: "Soap never touches my face!"

Elizabeth has always worn some sort of head covering when she steps outside: an immaculately crisp hat for public events, a loose scarf on private walks. Culture historian Peter Conrad sees it as a subliminal message of Queenship, a roundabout way to permanently wear the semblance of a crown at all times. Even when bareheaded, Elizabeth's "tightly permed white hair," he says, takes on the vision of an "adamantine helmet." The ubiquity of her headpieces, however, are a bit more pragmatic than that. Along with the parasols she occasionally carries, the Queen is simply doing her best to shade herself from the sun. A lifetime of doing so has been instrumental in preserving the radiance she was born with. "I need to keep out of the sun," she told Prince Philip during a visit to the Great Barrier Reef in the 1950s. Lolloping about in the intense equatorial flares himself, Philip barked from the water, "Do come in . . . You are a premature grandmother!" To figure out who ultimately won the argument is easy; only look at the rampant sun damage on Philip's face today. Another royal who threw caution to the solar winds was Princess Margaret. Her biannual beach-bum holidays on the Caribbean island of Mustique, beginning in the 1960s, did her Teutonic complexion no favors. Eventually "her skin leathered to an unroyal shade of bacon," says journalist Karen Heller.* These were just the sort of "weathering" activities the Queen has purposefully avoided, holidaying far north of the equator in Scotland for good measure. The precautions have paid off. Back in 1953 Cecil Beaton captured Elizabeth in his famous coronation photograph, looking like Snow White incarnate. Age has added its inevitable creases, but the canvas is still as snowy as ever.

---

* Margaret, let's not forget, incurred the double whammy of accelerated aging: smoking like a chimney. Lighting her first cigarette in bed, she could puff through 60 in a day, rarely breaking for meals. People spoke of being *kippered* during dinners with her. "When we started to eat, she lit a ciggie and then continued to chainsmoke, lighting one ciggie off another, throughout the meal," recalled a fellow diner. Margert had her smoking standards, of course, because she *was* Princess Margaret: one being her signature tortoise-shell cigarette holder (slightly less long than Cruella de Vil's), the other—never allowing the common rabble to light a smoke for her. "You don't light my cigarette, dear," she'd say to those who overestimated their royal intimacy. "Oh no, you're not that close."

Now a quick word about those creases: For a woman in her nineties, they are nowhere near as harsh or drawn as they could be. The result is based on a preventative measure, barely perceptible over time, and certainly not found in any expensive face cream. Elizabeth has simply put on a little weight as she has aged. Not a total pork out, obviously, just enough to soften and slightly plump her natural features. In doing so, she has altogether avoided the usual gaunt look of the elderly. A tactic likely inspired by the Queen Mother. Contrary to Wallis Simpson, who famously opined that a woman could never be too rich or too thin, the Queen Mother always felt that a little fullness in the cheeks was sort of nice, especially in the metaphorical mummy of the nation. Others did too. "She wasn't slim and chic and brittle (as 'Queen Wallis' would have been)," writes biographer Gyles Brandreth. "She was soft and round, regal yet real, classy but comfortable and comforting." It also made her look rosier and refreshed as she zoomed past her hundredth birthday. Becoming pleasingly plump made her more pleasing to look at. In contrast, thinner-is-a-winner Wallis (dying at 89) only grew more and more skeletal as she aged. All perfectly aligned with what British comedian Miranda Hart fantastically calls the "Fat Don't Crack" theory, an "anti-aging skincare" always guaranteed to "turn back the clock," she says, "based around a theory . . . that the skin of ever-so-slightly-chubby people does actually generally look rather nice."

If you're still skeptical, have a gander at Prince Philip, who has clearly *lost* weight in recent years. He looks every bit his old age. His cheeks are sunken and his skin is stretched over an increasingly prominent skull: features which epitomize the familiar look of frailty among the longer lived.* The tendency to gradually lose weight is one of the lesser-known side effects of living into one's eighties and beyond. Which is why a little buffer weight is medically advisable for seniors—particularly against falls, digestive problems, loses of appetite and unexpected hospital visits. Paradoxically, "the BMI curve shifts to the right as you age," explains

---

* Prince Philip, alas, has a teensy issue with weight, both on himself and on others. While inspecting a new spacecraft being built at Salford University, Philip asked a chubby thirteen-year-old boy if he'd like to travel on it one day. "Yes," said the boy. "You'll have to lose a bit of weight first," chided Philip.

Barbara Nicklas, professor of internal medicine at Wake Forest School of Medicine, "meaning higher weight is better in older age." A finding supported by the ongoing "90+ Study" out of the University of California, Irvine—one of the largest ongoing medical studies of seniors in the world. "It turns out that the best thing to do as you age is to at least maintain or even gain weight," concludes Claudia Kawas, a lead researcher on the project. "It's not good to be skinny when you're old." Neither does it seem to suit the people of Britain, who plainly prefer their Queens softer around the edges. Consider the wildly different reaction when the Australian artist Rolf Harris rolled out his portrait of Elizabeth in 2006. Depicting a comfortable-looking Queen with a bit of reassuring padding around the middle, it was the antidote the country needed after the Lucian Freud fiasco.

And yet, Elizabeth would never have sat for the controversial grandson of Sigmund Freud if vanity had any hold on her personality. Quite the contrary. Her courtiers say she rarely looks at herself in mirrors, will only do so to check that everything is in place and certainly doesn't spend time goggling. "She [has] little patience for gazing at herself in mirrors," says Sally Bedell Smith. "Vain preening [is] alien to her nature." She gets her hair done once a week. Margaret often got hers done twice a day. And though always exquisitely turned out, Elizabeth has really "never cared a fig" for clothes, as her governess once observed. She has never shown a hint of cleavage in her outfits and has kept the hemline of her dresses respectfully below the knee since 1952. She avoided the high shoulder pads of the 1980s and the miniskirt of the 1960s. Princess Diana might have felt the need, as one of her stylists observed, "to transform and transform until she found her true self," but the Queen's look has always been timeless and, as an important corollary, symbolically stable. Which has also meant aging in a timeless way too. The nips and tucks of plastic surgeons have never come near the Queen's visage. Her only facelift has been the "Windsor facelift" of a Hermès scarf tied around her chin while out walking, notes journalist Hannah Betts. "Yet there is something incredibly beautiful in the lack of vanity with which Her Majesty has aged: frank, unapologetic." Aging naturally has ensured that her iconic image has become a record, a living archive of accumulated experience and vast wisdom, not an artificial rewind of lessons hard-won. Like the Queen Mother once said to a photographer who suggested retouching a picture to smooth out her wrinkles, "I would not like to feel I had lived all these years without having anything to show for it."

This attitude is philosophically world's away from her Tudor namesake, Elizabeth I, who spent her last years on earth hiding behind a "Mask of Youth" (pitifully caking her face with toxic quantities of white lead). But today's Elizabeth believes that true *ageless* beauty is when you let age honestly speak for itself. "Take kindly the counsel of the years, gracefully surrendering the things of youth," admonished the poet Max Ehrmann. It was, the Queen said, one of the deeper lessons the American Revolutionary War taught to all subsequent monarchs across the pond. Speaking on the 1976 bicentennial celebration in Philadelphia, "as the direct descendant of King George III," she said that the Founding Fathers taught Britain and herself "a very valuable lesson." Specifically, "to know the right time, and the manner of yielding what is impossible to keep."

JUBILEE ME

OR RULE #21—LIFE GETS
BETTER AFTER 80

I am easier with myself these days, more forgiving, more content.
I have learned, for example, that there is life after cellulite.

—THE DUCHESS OF YORK

f you can hold out, there's one royal tradition worth waiting for. A mere hundred years, to be precise. Beginning in 1917 King George V sent congratulatory telegrams to every subject in the realm who had ripened to the venerable age of 100. That year, 24 centenarians received a bicycle-delivered message from the Palace that read: "His Majesty's hope that the blessings of good health and prosperity may attend you during the remainder of your days." Tastefully adorned cards have since replaced telegrams, and the birthday message has become a tad more modern, but the tradition continues. Elizabeth sends over a thousand cards every year with the help of a "centenarian team" at Whitehall, which keeps tabs on the oldest of the old throughout the country.* The cards have become cherished mementos of *jubilee* to

---

* Like every other centenarian, the Queen Mother received the royal greeting from the postman on her one-hundredth birthday in 2000. The only difference: it was signed "Lilibet" and her equerry opened the envelop with a flourish, using the tip of his sword in place of a letter opener.

those who receive them, a regal reminder to "shout for joy" in old age, as the Latin *jubilare* proclaims. They are emblematic of the Queen's belief that there is *more* to celebrate, not less, as the years mount up. It's a massively different message from the one delivered by popular culture. Namely, youths are "hot," elders are not—a culture where millennials stay "relevant" by getting Botox injections in their twenties. FOA (fear of aging) is nothing new, of course. Even Shakespeare's genius couldn't imagine the *last age of man* as anything beyond a fatalistic tragedy, a steady loss of one's bodily bits, a devolution of "sans teeth, sans eyes, sans taste, sans everything." Mildly less depressing is Dylan Thomas's poetic battle cry of the elderly, advising old sots everywhere to curse the coming darkness with their tennis-ball-tipped walkers, to "rage, rage against the dying of the light."

To appreciate how the Queen regards such bleak prospects for the future, one need only remember how she responded to the time T. S. Eliot came to the Palace for a private reading of his lugubrious poem "The Waste Land." As Eliot droned on about age and ruination, Elizabeth "got the giggles." The curve of her life has mercifully proved the stereotype wrong. The Queen hasn't slumped under the gravitas of old age, becoming harder and unhappier with the passing years. She has grown lighter and more full of life: doing, saying and enjoying things today that her middle-aged self wouldn't have freely countenanced. She veritably "blossomed" in her late seventies, notes biographer Sally Bedell Smith, recording how in 2003 Elizabeth was thrilled at the prospect of attending a birthday party at a London nightclub—something she hadn't done since her twenties. "Never have I seen anyone have such a good time," said a fellow partygoer. Telling as much to the dean of St. Alban's Abbey the following day, Elizabeth spotted another guest from the party, gleefully explaining to the rector that "[he] and I were in a nightclub last night till half past one." The same year Elizabeth held a dinner party at St. James's Palace for a group of Grenadier Guards who, on the occasion, were entertaining Elizabeth with boisterously loud jokes. The noise drifted up to the Queen's comptroller, Malcolm Ross, whose private apartment lay just above the dining room. Malcolm telephoned to complain about the lateness of the hour, oblivious to the fact that his boss was doing most of the partying below. When his complaint was passed on to Elizabeth, she replied, "Oh tell Malcolm not to be so silly."

In this regard Elizabeth has morphed very much into her mother, who was, by all accounts, *born* for old age. "Things are much more fun past eighty," the Queen Mother liked to say. "I am only just beginning to know what I like . . . & it is very exciting indeed." Piffling the fact that 49 was the average life expectancy for women of her generation, she discovered untapped reservoirs of strength as the years progressed. In 1980, surprising herself by how easily she traversed a bumpy patch of ground on the Frogmore estate, she wrote to Elizabeth: "I always think of how TIRED I felt, pottering down the hill with Granny & Grandpapa! Curiously enough, I don't feel half as tired at 79 as I did at 28!!" Psychologically she loosened up as well. Her relaxed outlook on life could have been mistaken for a college freshman. Especially the night when her former equerry, Jamie Lowther-Pinkerton, invited the remnants of his stag party back to his room at Clarence House (an oasis of free booze), forgetting the fact that the Queen Mother, in her eighties, was in residence and needed to get an early start for Trooping the Colour ceremony the next day. "The Private Secretary [eyed] me darkly," in the morning, Pinkerton recalls. But as he helped the Queen Mother into her carriage, she simply asked, "'Did you have a party here last night, Jamie?' I stared at my boots and mumbled, 'Ma'am, I'm terribly sorry. I hope we didn't disturb you,' knowing full well we had. 'I'm so glad to see the place being properly used,' Her Majesty sparked, hopping into the carriage."

Historian Lucy Worsley believes that Queen Victoria, for all her physical wobbles and weight gain, "became her best self in old age" too. The younger, glamorous versions of Victoria might get most of the limelight these days, but "only in maturity did she come out of the shadow of her husband's domineering personality, to emerge imperious, eccentric and really rather magnificent," says Worsley. Another respectable ripener, George III, went from being widely derided as a foreign German import at the start of his reign to gaining unprecedented reverence as his life lengthened to the then impressive age of 81 (and that was *despite* his battle with bipolar disorder). Prince Charles has become, if not exactly lovable, then certainly much more likable in his seventies.

Camilla is rapidly gaining ground too. Time hides a multitude of indis-
cretions, and "Britain as a whole tends to like its monarchs better as they
age," says Jeremy Paxman.

＊

Indeed the over-the-hill assumption of aging—as an inevitable *decline* in
well-being—is completely groundless. Time and again, social scientists
have found that the world's happiest, most satisfied people aren't in their
twenties, per the usual assumption, but in their eighties. A phenomenon now recognized as the "U-bend of life" shows that while most
people tend to experience a well-being "high" around young adulthood,
which dips and plateaus in middle age, they start on another ascent of
personal happiness in their seventies—an upward trajectory of inner
satisfaction that keeps on climbing into their eighties and beyond.
Currently, individuals in the 82–85 age bracket consistently rank higher
in life-enjoyment than eighteen-year-olds—a "U-bend" curve trending
worldwide, from western and eastern Europe, North and South America
and Asia. Yet with one fascinating stipulation: you have to *believe* it.
To believe, like the Queen Mother, that life *does* get better after 80.
People who have a negative perception of old age, seeing it as a spiral
down the u-bend of life's toilet, as it were, tend to live out a self-ful-
filling prophecy. Longitudinal studies at Yale University have shown
that younger individuals who dread getting old, believing their lives will
worsen and become useless as they age, were more likely to suffer from
serious heart problems, impaired memory and shorter life-spans than
people with a more positive outlook on old age. An astonishing seven
and a half years were added to the life expectancies of individuals who
simply *thought* about aging differently.

This is so strongly represented in the royal family, its members have
an unspoken rule about such things. Negative chatter and complaints
about aging are, quite literally, left unspoken. The same goes for the
minor illnesses and aches that come with old age. Unless they pose a
legitimate threat to life and limb, they are practically ignored. Hypochondriacs and malady-mongers are anathema in the House of Windsor.
If the Queen has long "radiated energy and robust good health," says
biographer Carolly Erickson, "it was in part because of an intolerant

attitude towards illness. Illness was not allowed in her world, either in herself or others. Insofar as possible, it was ignored." The occasional cold is treated, at best, as a minor inconvenience. "She has a theory that you carry on working and your cold gets better," a cousin of the Queen explains. When a physical inconvenience cannot be ignored, like the time the Queen Mother needed an operation to dislodge a fishbone caught in her throat, a mixture of levity and insouciance is always the correct Windsor response. Shrugging off her throat surgery, the Queen Mother (being a keen angler) merely noted, "After all these years of fishing, the fish are having their revenge." Likewise, when she needed a blood transfusion to correct a severe iron deficiency, Prince Charles preferred to mark the occasion with a congratulatory quip: "It was wonderful to see Your Majesty . . . with your iron constitution so comprehensively re-ironed." And when Elizabeth came down with the chicken pox at the awkward age of 45, she agreed to her confinement but insisted on referring to the illness as a "ridiculous disease." The Queen's ability to downplay the occasional bodily disorder is now such a firmly established trait, Peter Morgan included the following exchange in his royal-inspired play *The Audience*. Attempting to sympathize with Elizabeth after she has made an uncharacteristic slipup, Prime Minister John Major (unwisely) uses the crutch of illness:

> MAJOR: You were unwell that day.
> ELIZABETH: It was unconscionable. What I said. How
>   I behaved.
> MAJOR: You had the flu.
> ELIZABETH: I crossed the line. It was unforgiveable.
> MAJOR: You had a temperature.
> ELIZABETH: Cold.
> MAJOR: It was flu. The equerry made it quite clear . . .
> ELIZABETH: It was a cold!!

Traces of Stoicism doubtlessly underpin the habit, but it's also generational. The Windsors are a time capsule of a world that once thought along similar lines. Writing in the late 1930s, the memoirist Flora Thompson recalled the England of her childhood: "Such people at that time did not look for or expect illness, and there were not as many patent medicine advertisements then as now to teach them to search for symptoms of minor ailments in themselves." Even aspirin was regarded "as a dangerous drug," to the Queen Mother, said her niece Margaret Rhodes. "Her idea for curing a bad cold was a bracing walk in a stiff breeze across rugged terrain. It invariably worked!" As the Queen Mother herself would remind friends, "If you ignore illness it will go away."* The attitude made her amazingly resilient to the physical setbacks of old age. The press was always surprised at the speed in which she bounced back from surgeries, either after her two hip replacements in her nineties or when she fell and broke her collarbone at age 100. Only a few short weeks of recovery would pass before she was out of bed again, fulfilling her royal obligations. "She seemed indestructible," says royal chronicler Brian Hoey. Far more indestructible than Princess Margaret, who stubbornly kept plopping herself in a wheelchair in her late sixties (after badly scalding her feet in a hot bath). More than a year later, Margaret showed no signs or interest in gaining back full mobility. In one embarrassing scene of premature frailty, she quickly commandeered a wheelchair reserved for her mother—30 years her senior—during the elder's centenarian celebration. "Get out! That's meant for Mummy!" Elizabeth was heard to say on such occasions, perhaps angriest at the fact that Margaret appeared to be physically giving up far too soon. In two years she would be gone.

※

Willing oneself to longevity might not be as far-fetched as it sounds. In fact, it may very well be the ultimate placebo. Dan Buettner's global investigation of longevity specifically touched on the powerful component of optimism in individuals who reach well into their nineties and beyond, finding that "people who think they're going to live longer

---

* A lesson for all the hypochondriacs out there: Dwelling too much on what could physically go wrong in your body might actually make you sicker in the long run, according to a large study out of Norway. Studying levels of "health anxiety" (hypochondria) in over 7,000 subjects, it found that people who worried about their health were 70 percent more likely to develop heart disease than people who brushed off the occasional ache or pain.

actually do." Pessimistic grumps, on the other hand, were significantly absent from the longest-lived people groups around the world. An observation reinforced by a recent study out of Boston University of Medicine, showing that optimistic thinkers are more likely to experience "exceptional longevity" than their curmudgeonly counterparts. Only consider the Queen Mother's cheery pronouncement, after successfully recovering from an illness later in life: "I'm going to live to a hundred." She exceeded her goal by nearly two years.*

The Queen Mother's clothes were symbolic of this indomitable optimism. Normally some pastel shade of pink, blue or purple, they sartorially reflected the soft lens through which she viewed the act of aging itself. The outward fabric took on, what Prince Charles has called, her "effervescent enthusiasm for life." In the same way, Elizabeth has become what her wardrobe declares. She has naturally gravitated towards brighter clothes in the winter of her reign, choosing vibrant shades like daffodil yellow, periwinkle blue, lime green and lilac. They ostensibly help her stand out in a crowd, yes, but Queen Victoria was pretty visible, as well, in her frumpy black frocks. The queen of Hollywood, Elizabeth Taylor, had an intriguing theory about such things. She believed that people gradually aged into a look that reflected their inner spirit. "When you're young, sheer physical beauty can carry you along," she said. "As you get older, what you are begins to affect your looks. A sweet, tranquil character can erase lines and smooth a sagging chin. A

---

* The power of positive thinking may explain the royal family's historic trust in homeopathy. Treating an illness by taking very diluted doses of a natural substance that would induce the illness under normal circumstances—the gist of homeopathy—often amounts to little more than a placebo. But the Windsors have sworn by it since the days of Queen Victoria. If possible, Elizabeth always prefers to start with natural remedies before moving on to more mainstream drugs. Her sinus infections, for instance, have been treated with the homeopathic tincture of arsenic (heavily diluted) in Malvern water. Arnica tablets and ointments are readily administered at the Palace should anyone suffer a minor bruise. There's also hawthorn for high blood pressure and belladonna for sore throats. The Queen has equal faith in her more orthodox doctors, and serious conditions aren't experimented on in the same way. When Elizabeth heard that one of her stable hands had developed a brain tumor, her swift action to arrange the surgery to remove the growth saved the man's life.

selfish, hard personality can obliterate the most perfect features." If that is true, then the Queen has truly aged well. She smiles more nowadays and is "warmer, more approachable, and more relaxed" than ever before, says Sally Bedell Smith.

＊

The grim alternative has always been before her, to harden and emotionally calcify over the years, a path chosen by the geriatric grouches in her family tree, like George V. He might have begun the tradition of sending out birthday greetings to centenarians, but there was little to celebrate about the way he personally aged. George V rotted more than ripened, becoming an angry old man that few people, save his favorite grandchild, Lilibet, actually wanted to be around. Increased isolation was Princess Margaret's lot too. She regressed to such infuriating levels of immaturity as she grew older, her husband started leaving vicious notes around the house for her to find, including the unforgettable, "Twenty Four Reasons Why I Hate You." One of her many tragedies was always feeling uncomfortable with her age. "I was born too late," she complained as a girl, whenever Elizabeth took part in activities Margaret was too young for. As an older woman, she bemoaned being born too soon. A mismatch she tried to correct with horrendous results: sometimes with liaisons with stupid young men, sometimes by knocking back too many whiskeys, but mainly through embarrassing displays of teenage-style angst—"growing more and more temperamental, alternately moody and fractious, like a refractory child," says Carolly Erickson. Margaret ultimately failed to appreciate the gifts she had when she had them.

Because most importantly, U-bends of life require gratitude. "Count your blessings!" was the Queen Mother's dependable antidote against the glums. So much so, when William Shawcross compiled her personal letters for publication, the book's title chose itself: *Counting One's Blessings*. Gratitude kept her in the moment, finding joy in the least occasions of life. When she received a set of large bath towels for her 101st birthday—a simple gift for a woman who had everything—she told the sender how "heavenly" it was that, at last, she could now wrap her entire body up in fluffy luxury. "She turned even the most tedious occasions into a party," remembered Margaret Rhodes, affirming the accuracy of an article in *The Times* that noted how the Queen Mother could attend a dull charity function or lay "a foundation stone as though she [had] discovered a new and delightful way of spending an afternoon." Her life truly exemplified the words of a lovely old slogan once popular in Britain:

Life ain't all you want,
But it's all you 'ave;
So 'ave it;
Stick a geranium in yer 'at
An' be 'appy.

You could choose otherwise, certainly. But as the Queen Mother liked to point out, "tomorrow you might be run over by a big red bus!"*

---

* Few proved the point more pitifully than that other queen of Hollywood, Marilyn Monroe. When she was 36, Monroe was horrified by the prospect of turning 40, often crying buckets in her dressing room when she discovered a new, barely perceptible wrinkle on her face. "She was so depressed about those wrinkles!" remembered her hairstylist Sydney Guilaroff, who consoled Marilyn's fears about aging, reassuring her that "she looked fine," just three days before she died.

THE MARMITE THEORY

OR RULE #22—STRETCH YOUR CROWN

Happiness . . . is neither virtue nor pleasure
nor this thing or that, but simply growth.
We are happy when we are growing.

—JOHN BUTLER YEATS

Where would future monarchs be without their wizened mentors? King Arthur had Merlin. Elizabeth had Henry Marten. The eccentric 66-year-old vice-provost of Eton College, known for nervously sucking on his handkerchiefs, keeping a pet raven in his study and nibbling on lumps of sugar secretly pulled from his pocket, Marten seemed an unlikely fit for educating a thirteen-year-old girl on the finer points of Queenship. Absentmindedly forgetting that he was speaking to a girl and not a classroom of male Etonians, he would occasionally refer to Elizabeth as "Gentlemen." Yet in 1938 Henry Marten began imparting lessons to Elizabeth she has depended on for decades. Twice a week she sat in his study at Eton, where the books appeared to grow upward from the floor like stalagmites in a cave. There the long history of the British monarchy was rolled out before her. At a superficial angle, it rather looked like *1066 and All That* (a comic history book published a few years earlier), which posited royal history as one big hodgepodge of "good things" and "bad

211

things." But Henry Marten didn't see it that way. Change was history's one constant, and he believed the monarchy's ability to adapt to it was one of its greatest secrets of survival. It was Constitutional History 101. The Kings and Queens who adapted to change were "good things." Those who remained stubbornly set in their ways were not. Elizabeth's reign would be no different. Her success, if she could pull it off, would be to provide the semblance of continuity while stretching the Crown around a constantly evolving world. Otherwise known as "the Marmite theory of monarchy."

Coined at the cusp of the new millennium by the Queen's private secretary Robin Janvrin, it took its inspiration from the jars of Marmite commonly found in British kitchens for over a hundred years. The salty yeast paste (slash food spread, slash tar in a jar, slash don't ask) seemingly hasn't changed for generations. For most people, a jar of Marmite today, with its familiar red, green and yellow logo, looks identical to the ones their grandparents bought. In actuality, the jar has undergone significant changes over time—a marketing magic trick based on slow, barely perceptible adaptations over many years. All along the jars have been gradually improving without ever sacrificing the nostalgia customers have relied upon. To survive, "the monarchy needed to change the same way," says biographer Sally Bedell Smith, "incrementally over time, small steps rather than large steps, so people were reassured that the institution was staying the same while adapting." Britain still liked the permanence of the royal family, yes, but it didn't want its members permanently pickled in aspic either. Balancing the two has arguably been the trickiest job of every monarch since the tumultuous days of Magna Carta. And Elizabeth has not only pulled it off admirably, she has done it on a bigger scale than any of her predecessors.

＊

In 1957 an obscure magazine editor named John Grigg published the soon-to-be notorious article "The Monarchy Today," outlining his recommendations to modernize the monarchy for the twentieth century. The only way ahead, as Grigg saw it, was for the ancient institution to become more egalitarian and open with its people. Elizabeth might have been born into a world where Britain's Kings and Queens didn't smile too frequently, lest they break the spell of sovereignty, but that would no longer suit a more democratic world. Not being the meekest of chaps (he wasn't afraid to say that the Queen sounded like "a priggish schoolgirl" when she spoke), Grigg's analysis was widely denounced as the ravings of a deluded progressive.* Being more accessible to her ordinary subjects, more "classless," as Grigg proposed, seemed shockingly avant-garde for an institution allegedly based on the tribal magic of a chieftain who doesn't emerge too frequently from her royal hut—and who certainly doesn't let the hoi polloi inside. The real shock, however, is how carefully Elizabeth listened, taking Grigg's recommendations for what they were, "loyal and constructive criticism," and gradually enacting practically all of his well-meant advice. And more so.

She was the first monarch to allow the world inside the inner sanctum of Buckingham Palace, first by turning the Christmas broadcast into a live television event, previously shrouded behind the mystery of radio waves, then by allowing BBC filmmakers to capture the Windsors at home. The resulting 1969 documentary, *Royal Family*, with its quaint scenes of barbecues at Balmoral and jaunts with the Queen to a village shop to buy candy for Prince Edward, seemed as radical and futuristic as the moon landing that year, says biographer Robert Hardman. So too was her historic decision to abolish the elite pageantry of the Season. Once a gathering of aristocratic debutantes at Buckingham Palace (part dizzying parade of eligible young ladies in white silk dresses, part open season for husband hunting), it had occurred, every year, since the days of George III. In its place, Elizabeth began the new, more inclusive tradition of summer garden parties, welcoming thousands to the Palace from all socioeconomic walks of life. The once stringent protocols of curtseys and bows have likewise been relaxed under Elizabeth's reign. The Queen even speaks differently today from how she was raised to speak. Her cut-glass accent, her "priggish schoolgirl" voice, has gradually lost

---

* Grigg received a metaphorical slap from the press and a real one from Philip Kinghorn Burbidge. "I felt it was up to a decent Briton to show resentment," said Burbidge, a 64-year-old ex-soldier and member of a staunch society of fellow Loyalists, who tracked down Grigg on a London street and soundly cuffed him across the face, saying, "Take that from the League of Empire Loyalists!" A pretty stupendous line, and one I really must insist on if anyone cuffs me.

its aristocratic clink, becoming smoother and rounder and much more relatable over the years.

On top of it all, "the Queen has seen a staggering amount of change" she has had no control over, says political commentator Andrew Marr. A differential press has been replaced by a mob of prying sensationalists, a substantial empire under her father into a patchy Commonwealth, a supportive Parliament into a hypocritical body of spendthrifts who, if they could, would question the cost of the tissue the Queen uses to sneeze into. So much has changed, it's often said that if history's two famous Georges came back to life—George III and George Washington—the British George wouldn't be able to cope with the monumental changes at Buckingham Palace, whereas the American George would still feel quite at home in the White House. The top job in the iconic land of progress, ironically, has stayed more static than the top job of Britain.* The greatest leaps of change have not only occurred in Elizabeth's lifetime, they have occurred at the latter end of it—a time when change *should* be the most difficult to accept. "Yet bizarrely," says Andrew Marr, the Queen "has emerged from all this [change] not shredded and diminished, but strengthened." One could say she has coped so well because she has aged according to the Marmite theory too.

※

Elizabeth has never stopped learning, listening to criticism or being open to new experiences. "Change has become a constant," she remarked on her fiftieth anniversary on the throne in 2002. "Managing it has become an expanding discipline. The way we embrace it defines our future." The Queen loves her daily routines, the way her year unfolds in predictable patterns, but she has also seen the consequences of complacency, when royals get into a rut. Her grandfather, George V, was so afraid of the social and political changes sweeping post–World War I Britain,

---

* George III would feel more comfortable in the Oval Office today too, where the executive powers of the US presidency were modeled on those of an eighteenth-century British King, with a few more executive powers thrown in for good measure. "We elect a king for four years," observed Abraham Lincoln's secretary of state, "and give him absolute power with certain limits, which after all he can interpret for himself." No truer words.

he steeped royal life in the formaldehyde of his Victorian childhood, waging "a private war with the twentieth century," said his eldest son. Painted fingernails, jazz music and boyish haircuts on women were as discombobulating for him as finding one of his favorite chairs or hairbrushes out of place. His "hatred of change was almost pathological," writes biographer Sarah Bradford. "His short temper would explode if a housemaid happened to move a piece of furniture from its accustomed place." He could never have handled the "reforms" Elizabeth has navigated so smoothly in recent years—paying taxes, unprecedented budget slashes, connecting with her subjects via social media, visiting mosques and Hindu temples, the ordination of women in the Church of England, drastic reductions in Britain's military forces and the impending likelihood of Scottish independence.

And to think, the Queen Mother once found it difficult to accept the most minor modernizations around the Palace—like her fuss over the de-wigging of royal footmen or the abandonment of hand-delivered messages in favor of an updated intercom system. Elizabeth, however, has remained remarkably "plastic" as she has aged, to borrow a term from neuroscience. She has kept on bending and stretching and extending her mind to accommodate new ideas and new ways of thinking, as she herself has admitted, at an "accelerating pace over these years." Neuroplasticity is what makes the brains of children so elastic, and it's the hallmark of successful aging too. Flexible brains stay fresher.* Graceful acceptance of change and criticism has kept the Queen so mentally agile over the years, there's little chance now that her worst-case scenario will ever come to fruition.

That is, there is technically one proviso to the Queen's blank refusal

---

* By far one of the more promising medical discoveries in recent years has been debunking the conventional view that adult brains are rigidly "hardwired" and unable to change past a certain age. In actuality, learning new skills can keep "rewiring" the brain's neuropathways well into old age. Spectacularly demonstrated in 1996, when an optimistic George Dawson, aged 98, decided to right decades of wrong and finally get the education his poor upbringing in rural Texas denied him. Unable, at the start, to even read his ABCs, Dawson returned to school, became a stellar student at the age of 101, and was soon writing a best-selling book about the experience, titled *Life Is So Good.*

to abdicate in old age. As she told her cousin Margaret Rhodes, she will never prematurely pass on the crown "unless I get Alzheimer's or have a stroke," at which point Prince Charles would step in as acting King *in loco parentis*, creating a constitutional Regency while the Queen slips quietly into semiretirement. The historic precedent was theoretically established by George III, when he started losing his royal marbles in old age and doing undignified things like, allegedly, shaking hands with an oak tree in Windsor Great Park, thinking it was the king of Prussia. Filling the sanity vacuum, his widely unpopular son became Prince Regent for nine years—a period more remembered for the romantic novels of Jane Austen than the constitutional crisis caused by the King's cognitive decline. But imagine the dismal prospect of Prince Charles as Regent today, and you can better appreciate the historic dilemma. Regencies aren't romantic; they are a necessary evil. Luckily it's only a far-fetched speculation nowadays, as there appears to be little chance of a new Regency period under Elizabeth's watch. She came out of the womb, as her mother observed, "as sharp as a needle" and has resiliently remained so.

※

Like those ever-evolving jars of Marmite, the Queen has been impercep-tibly improving her noggin for decades—especially in her free time, a habit she picked up from her grandmother.

Queen Mary never enjoyed "resting" in the conventional sense of the term, preferring Lord Crewe's view that "the best form of relaxation is to do some other kind of work." Resting for Queen Mary meant reading, or being read to by one of her ladies-in-waiting, particularly when she was sitting for hours while having her portrait painted. "In either case," said her biographer James Pope-Hennessy, resting "meant using and improving her mind." Elizabeth feels the same. She watches television sparingly, preferring the radio instead, and fills her scant leisure time with her favorite brainteaser: crossword puzzles. She completes the *Daily Telegraph*'s two crosswords every day (without using a thesaurus, which she says is cheating) and is rumored to keep a few emergency puzzles in her handbag at all times. She can reputedly polish off *The Time*'s puzzle in an impressive four minutes. On holidays, the Queen flexes her cerebral muscles further with ridiculously large jigsaw puzzles. Sometimes stretching to 10,000 pieces, a puzzle on the round baize-covered table at Sandringham is as much a fixture of the winter season with the royals as a Christmas tree. Journalist Jeremy Paxman tried tackling one of these interlocking behemoths at Sandringham a few years ago and found the endeavor "impossible"—"the pieces are all dark green or black and there is no accompanying box-top to show even which way up the final picture should be." Despite "the collective brainpower" of others, he admitted, he only "managed to assemble about twenty pieces" before he left. Perhaps this is not the time to remind Paxman that the Queen has been observed successfully matching up the pieces, with her back turned, while carrying on a conversation with guests.*

Elizabeth has such a puzzle-oriented brain, she excelled in the unlikely skill (for a princess) of auto mechanics during the war. At eighteen, just as others her age were also mucking in to defeat Hitler, she trained with the Auxiliary Territorial Service, wearing grease-stained coveralls and popping the bonnets of lorries to fiddle her way around the puzzling complexities of the combustion engine. Skills that have remained with her to this day, along with the claim that she can still change a carburetor with her eyes closed. Her cousin Margaret Rhodes believed Elizabeth gradually learned to approach the engine of monarchy in much the same way. With so many demands on her mental attention—niggling matters of state, entertaining foreign dignitaries, family affairs—she has had to develop "a compartmentalized brain, with lots of boxes," said Rhodes. "She can appear frightfully jolly while a constitutional question is going on in another part of her mind." An affinity for puzzles might also explain the Queen's reported fondness for detective stories and for speaking in riddles. More importantly, puzzles seem to

---

* Puzzles don't have a monopoly on keeping the mind sharp—all sorts of problem-solving exercises can slow and prevent cognitive decline—but puzzles, especially word puzzles, do seem to tap into a very primal part of the human brain. Word games and riddles were "among the most important precursors of systematic knowledge," says psychologist Mihaly Csikszentmihalyi. "In the most ancient cultures, the elders of the tribe would challenge each other to contests in which one person sang a text filled with hidden references, and the other person had to interpret the meaning encoded in the song."

be doing an excellent job at keeping her brain remarkably inquisitive in old age—a hugely important mental faculty which tends to atrophy as people get older. It's part of the Queen's job to constantly pose questions to prime ministers, to cabinet officials, to honorable guests at cocktail receptions or to ordinary folks during her walkabouts. But there is oftentimes a real, almost childlike curiosity behind Elizabeth's questions about life, extending far beyond the two stereotypically drab queries the press give her credit for: "Have you come far?" and "What is it that you do?" Take her brilliant question to a group of medical students while touring a hospital in 2002—"Why does one have wax in one's ears?" None of the doctors-in-training could tell her.

The lack of a university degree has never stopped Elizabeth from constantly learning. In fact, it has probably accelerated it. There have always been intellectual snobs who demean her academic underachievements. Peter Morgan, writer of Netflix's *The Crown*, repeated the trite view, describing the Queen as a "countryside woman of limited intelligence." Good grief, everyone's intelligence is limited in some way. But if Elizabeth has felt the need to constantly catch up, it has only benefited her in the long run, turning her into "an extraordinarily shrewd and perceptive observer of the world," to quote Tony Blair. The Queen has such a phenomenal memory, a capacity to absorb information and government documents faster than her red boxes can be delivered, Lord David Owen, the former Labour foreign secretary, is convinced that Elizabeth would "have gotten a first-class degree if she'd gone to university, I have no doubt about that." Very few of the intelligentsia could handle the Queen's job. Or be able to remember, particularly in old age, the vast amount of political, social and cultural details Elizabeth has needed to retain in order to be a living database of information that young prime ministers can consult at need. Nor could they repeatedly wow their subjects by stupendous feats of recall . . .

In 1953 Nancy Byrne was just another musician in the Dunedin Ladies' Brass Band of Palmerston, New Zealand—a group which among hundreds of others, performed for the Queen during her first Commonwealth tour. Thirty-seven years later, at a garden party in New Zealand, Nancy Byrne was introduced to the Queen again, though hardly expecting a shadow of remembrance to pass across Elizabeth's face.

But being "overwhelmed by the occasion," Nancy recalled, a bystander blurted out to the Queen, "'Oh, but Nancy met you when you came to Palmerston last time.' And the Queen looked at me and said, 'Ladies' brass band.' 'Yes, Ma'am,' I replied." Encounters like that have done more to humanize the monarchy than anything else. And a memory like that, alas for Prince Charles, has all but obliterated his chances of becoming a Regent anytime soon. Your mother is in full possession of her wits, good sir, as Jane Austen might say.

LONDON BRIDGE

OR RULE #23—DIE LIKE YOU LIVED IT

In my end is my beginning.
—MARY, QUEEN OF SCOTS

For all the bizarre reactions to Princess Diana's death in 1997, few things were freakier than the BBC's quick response. They almost seemed prepared for it. Faster than the British public could pronounce *Pitié-Salpêtrière*—the hospital where the princess died—broadcasters at the BBC were airing polished interviews with royal experts, announcing the tragedy in perfectly delivered tones of solemnity and rolling out condensed bios of her life, segmented by expertly edited obituary footage. It was as if they had been practicing for the event for months, if not years, in advance. Indeed they had.

It wasn't because Diana was particularly reckless at the latter end of her life. She was, of course, but she wasn't singled out. Every top royal in Britain gets the same treatment. Death rehearsals are a fundamental fact of life for the Windsors. Behind the scenes, the BBC prepared so long for Diana's "unexpected" exit, they were ready for numerous eventualities, including the poignantly predictive scenario of her dying in a car crash on the M4 motorway. The Queen Mother's death was likewise rehearsed for years at the newsroom, usually on the mock premise that choking on a fish bone had done her in.* At one time, Prince Philip was postulated

---

* In reality, she died incredibly peacefully—on Easter Saturday 2002 in her bedroom at Royal

to putter out after being accidentally shot by his son Edward while out hunting. The BBC is nothing but not prepared for expiring royals. There's even RATS at the ready ("radio alert transmission system"), a cold war–era emergency alarm, primed to alert the wider media in the event of, as its nickname implies, a "royal [is] about to snuff it." But that's been hitherto reserved for the Big One: the Queen's death day.

The occasion will undoubtedly catch millions off guard, but Elizabeth has been preparing for it since the 1960s. Twice a year she has thought about and tweaked the details of a massive ten-day spectacle, her biggest yet, which she won't be present for. Involving the coordinated efforts of a dozen government departments, the army, police force and media heads, nothing has been left to chance. Nighttime rehearsals of her funeral procession along the streets of London are secretly practiced and perfected every year. The timing has been impeccably rehearsed, with the wheels of her cortège coming to a stop outside Westminster Hall just before Big Ben's tenor bell tolls. "The next great rupture in Britain's national life has, in fact, been planned to the minute," says journalist Sam Knight. A stock of headlines, stories and documentaries to accompany the event are already in place. Many in the press rehearse their announcements of Elizabeth's death every six months. *The Times* reportedly has eleven days of coverage already planned. Even radio stations in Britain are prepared to play a more somber selection of songs when the RATS alarm, one day, goes off.

The level of preparation has been unparalleled, but not entirely unprecedented. The Queen Mother's funeral was ongoingly planned for 22 years. Princess Margaret's day of reckoning was endlessly tweaked as well. "I am always altering the arrangements for my funeral," she told a friend. Queen Victoria chose the items she wanted buried alongside her almost 30 years in advance of the occasion. And Winston Churchill, who was practically a royal by adoption, summoned a committee

---

Lodge, Windsor. A cough and a chest infection (along with a heart broken by Princess Margaret's untimely death a month before) had weakened her body irrevocably. She had ample time, however, to say farewell to friends and hand out a few parting treasures. Her final words were quietly spoken to Elizabeth, sitting up beside her fireplace, before she breathed her last while being tenderly prayed over by her chaplain. She was 101 years and 238 days old.

of 31 people to discuss his ceremonial parting six years prior to his death, arrangements they code-named "Operation Hope Not." A bit too obvious for the Windsors, who have chosen more incognito code names for their final farewells. Based on various bridges throughout Britain, there was "Operation Tay Bridge" for the Queen Mother, "Forth Bridge" currently for Prince Philip, "Menai Bridge" for Prince Charles and "London Bridge" for the Queen. "London Bridge is down" is assumed to be the phrase by which the current prime minister will be quietly notified of Elizabeth's passing.

＊

So much death-talk amongst the living may sound strangely macabre to non-royal ears—downright "beastly" even, to use a favorite adjective of the Queen Mother's. Surely it's the here and now that should occupy our thoughts, not some hypothetical D-day a long way off. Like an inevitable visit from the dreaded in-laws, we prefer to get by by avoiding it. Our language about death is increasingly nonconfrontational. Once an unavoidable fixture of village life, cemeteries have been rebranded "Memorial Parks," displaced to the least frequented limits of cities and towns, their gravestones taking on the innocuous new identity of "markers." The dying are outsourced to hospitals; far less messy that way. And caskets, once placed in a familiar nook in a parlor at home, are now attended to at a comfortable distance, laid out nicely by complete strangers at professional funeral parlors. We've been getting so good at tuning out our collective death knell, over half of all American adults have avoided sitting down to hash out the details of their last will. We aren't technically afraid of death, as Woody Allen famously opined, we just don't want to be there when it happens.

Yet the irony is, by regularly avoiding the thought of death, we have robbed ourselves of one of the most powerful tools for building better lives. Because for all its foggy mysteries, death is the single biggest long-focus lens we have. It's the Hubble telescope of life, cutting through the confusing atmosphere of daily, petty, existential dramas to show us what existence is all about. The dying (if they are lucky) look through the lens most clearly, seeing life at a crystalline angle of awareness they have never experienced before. For many, however, the clarity can be too clear for comfort. Nearing his own death, Edward VIII looked back on the family, the country and the Crown he exchanged for his sexual infatuation with Wallis Simpson and finally realized the tremendous price he paid for it all: "What a waste! What a waste! What a waste!" were some of his last words on earth. Elizabeth I, who gloried in the accumulation of wealth throughout her life, counted those riches as nothing as she drew closer to death. More time was what she most wanted now. "All my possessions for a moment of time," she pleaded before passing. Though few end-of-life regrets are as hauntingly sad as the one by French writer Sidonie-Gabrielle Colette: "What a wonderful life I've had! I only wish I'd realized it sooner."

Now the big question, perhaps the biggest question of all: Should you wait for the end of your existence to experience what will likely be your most focused moment of all? The Queen doesn't think so. Regularly pondering her own death, seriously thinking about her funeral twice a year for over 60 years has been, as her courtiers have confirmed, "healthy and important" for the Queen. It has reminded her, as she puts it, "to take the long view" of life, to see herself as a passing steward, not an owner, of her royal treasures, to always put Crown and country before herself and to stay remarkably humble in a position of intrinsic haughtiness.* Death has reminded Elizabeth, in the blunt words of Michel de Montaigne, that "even on the most exalted throne in the world we are only sitting on our own bottom." She believes a good death is worth preparing for. She is in good company.

✳

Elizabeth's Christian faith, like every great religion, is layered with reminders that life can only be lived fully when we remember that it is limited. "So teach us to number our days, that we may apply our hearts unto wisdom," says the Psalmist. The Buddha similarly believed that

---

* Much of the Queen's earthly possessions are, in fact, on loan. Estimations of Elizabeth's wealth can be wildly exaggerated because they include priceless treasures like the Crown Jewels, artwork from the Royal Collection and the property value of Windsor Castle and Buckingham Palace. Instead these assets are owned by the British nation and are merely "held in trust" by the Queen during her lifetime. She can never sell them for a bit of ready cash.

death-thoughts were doorways to higher realms of mental clarity, coun-
seling that "of all mindfulness meditations, that on death is supreme."
The beauty and richness of Japanese art could likewise not exist without
the constant awareness of death, a concept known as *mono no aware*,
the melancholy of impermanence, the reality that all things—a flower,
a stream, a moonbeam, a life—are transient and therefore infinitely
precious. Western art once strongly reflected the belief. *Memento
mori*—reminders of deaths—were religiously incorporated into the
most beautiful paintings. Skulls were positioned near tulips, skeletons
lurked in the shadows of dinner parties. They were not meant to horrify
or depress but to wake up the artist and viewers from the dangerous
illusion of immortality. *Memento mori* means "remember that you will
die." Interestingly, the only portrait of Elizabeth I with a *memento mori*
beside her (where, like ominous page boys, Death and Father Time
flank an aging Queen) was painted seven years *after* her death. She never
tolerated such reminders of transience while living, or anything that
contradicted her delusion of eternal youth. Although one can't help but
feel that Gloriana would have suffered fewer inglorious regrets on her
deathbed if she had done so.

The ancient Stoics would have said she needed more *premeditatio
malorum* in her life—the ability to confront and calmly ponder its worst-
case scenarios before they happen—the ultimate worst, of course, being
death itself. Only by regularly visualizing our ends could we live out our
fullest potential. "Let us prepare our minds as if we'd come to the very
end of life," said Seneca. "Let us postpone nothing. Let us balance life's
books each day. . . . The one who puts the finishing touches on their life
each day is never short of time." People who ignore the inevitable, who
act as if they "were going to live ten thousand years," warned Marcus
Aurelius, were not only in for a nasty shock, they were likely frittering
away their remaining time in ways that, one day, they would deeply
regret. Backwards to front was the best way to approach one's book of
life, argued the Stoics, the only way to ensure that the chapter you are
writing now, if it is indeed your last, could be read with pride.*

---

* The Queen has the double advantage of actually living this reality. Her official biographer has
been watching everything from the sideline for decades, ready to publish the ninety-plus-year

Stephen Covey would go on to rediscover the wisdom of beginning "with the end in mind," famously identifying it as one of the "seven habits of highly effective people." By starting with the person you want to be remembered for, said Covey, "you can make certain that whatever you do on any particular day does not violate the criteria you have defined as supremely important, and that each day of your life contributes in a meaningful way to the vision you have of your life as a whole." Others simply refer to it as the Tombstone Test—arguably the most jolting of thought experiments. Namely, do your actions today reflect what you ultimately want inscribed on your tombstone? Do they get you closer or further from the eulogy you would like spoken at your funeral service? Knowing how you want to exit this world is crucial for determining how you want to live in it. If Princess Diana had taken more time to contemplate her future death, even at the apparently invincible age of 36, she would never have dated a reckless, cocaine-addicted playboy, jetted with him to Paris or got into an unfamiliar car the night that ended everything. Ironically, by casually ignoring her own mortality, she actually accelerated it. None of us can choose our expiration date, but our actions can have a dramatic effect on our shelf life. As one of the most highly effective people on the planet (Oprah Winfrey) has pointed out, "If this were the last day of your life, would you spend it the way you're spending today?"

The Queen Mother had a secret tombstone phrase which helped curate her answer. It was a simple line from the medieval mystic poet Julian of Norwich: "All shall be well, and all manner of things shall be well." It became "her personal philosophy," says biographer Elizabeth Longford, guiding her response in every crisis, from World War II to

---

narrative after her death. Eliminating as many awkward chapters as possible has doubtless been a huge motivator in the Queen's life. Though you can tap into the same motivation yourself. Researchers call it "autobiographical reasoning," the ability to look ahead and visualize the big themes of your own biography. How does what you're doing now contribute (or distract) from the story you *want* to read. If there are pitfalls along the way, will you climb out in the next chapter? "Always live your life with your biography in mind," advises the writer Marisha Pessl. "Naturally, it won't be published unless you have a Magnificent Reason, but at the very least you will be living grandly."

the scandalous breakdown of royal marriages in the 1990s. She wanted courage, calm and determined, to be her legacy—to be the stalwart image portrayed in one of her favorite newspaper clippings. It described her launching a battleship many years before: "On the dais stood the Queen, chatting to the bishop, and waving to the crowd. Suddenly—silently—she was in the sea, surrounded by a mass of broken wreckage." She wanted to be as buoyant as that battleship, someone who kept chugging courageously on through the disappointing wreckage of life. And by knowing how she wanted to be remembered, she lived just so. At the thanksgiving service marking her eightieth birthday, a massive banner was unfurled in St. Paul's Cathedral bearing the words of her self-perpetuating prophecy: "All shall be well, and all manner of things shall be well." Twenty-one years later, after she was gone, the words were still being used to sum up her legacy. Some in the press took to calling her "Mother Courage." It was testament to another truth held dear by her daughter the Queen: "The true measure of all our actions is how long the good in them lasts." A life well lived will always create a good which outlasts you.

Once upon a time, this idea was immortalized in an important doctrine of kingship. Every King or Queen of England, it was believed, was a mystically hybrid creature with two bodies: their physical body, which one day would die, and an immortal body impervious to time, age and decay. It was this incorruptible body, the magical spirit of kingship, that tied every past monarch of England together, migrating seamlessly from one rightful successor to the next in an unbroken chain of majesty. The sovereign of England, therefore, *technically* never dies. He or she is always the eternal embodiment of the once and future king.* Hence the requisite cry whenever the physical body of any sovereign passes

---

* Subsequently, the Royal Standard *never* flies at half-mast, even on the occasion of a monarch's death. To do so would signify the death of the monarchy itself—a crucial concept flagrantly ignored by the press after Diana's death. In attempts to deflect blame away from themselves, they turned the public's gaze on the one so-called "insensitive" building in London without a semi-hoisted flag, Buckingham Palace. Unfortunately, the public gullibly took the bait, forcing the Queen into an unprecedented compromise: flying the Union Jack at half-mast over the Palace instead.

away: "The King is dead, long live the King." Which better explains why Elizabeth is so partial to the imagery of the "bridge" when referring to her own death-day arrangements. Her funeral will be the bridge that connects us all to the next royal adventure.

※

When a life has dutifully lived out its full purpose, death is never a dead end. Bridges *always* continue on, linking the past to the future. British royals once related to the mythical imagery of the phoenix for the same reason; a bird that rose again from its own ashes reminded them that death was just the beginning, not the end, of their legacy. This is as true for Kings and Queens as it is for paupers, postmen, mechanics and stay-at-home moms. The anthropologist Ernest Decker called it having an "immortality project"—the heritage you will leave behind according to the life you have chosen to live. The Queen calls it thinking in terms of "if only"—not from the perspective of the past, "to look down a blind alley" full of regret, she says, but to look forward in the months, years and generations ahead "and say 'if only.'"

In the children's nursery rhyme, London Bridge might fall down, but it's instantly built up again, bigger and better than before. The foundations are strong. The future is secure. Whether Elizabeth is with us for ten more years or ten more minutes, everything she has represented, worked for, struggled against, gracefully conceded and helped to sustain will remain. In living well she has bridged death itself. And however long she is with us, come what may, we can always stand on that bridge and repeat the same heartfelt invocation that resounded at her coronation over 60 years ago. With thousands of triumphant voices proclaiming, *"God save Queen Elizabeth! Long live Queen Elizabeth! May the Queen live forever!*

WE'RE
BIGGER
THAN
WE'VE
EVER
DREAMED
AND
I'M IN
LOVE
WITH
BEING
QUEEN . . .

—Lorde, "Royals"

Appendix

THE 23 QUEEN BE'S

1. Be an undramatic eater
2. Be treatful with yourself
3. Be mannerly at mealtime
4. Be a self-transcendent drinker
5. Be limited by the freedom of order
6. Be courteous to others and concise with your time
7. Be poised and posturally powerful
8. Be devoted to your devoir
9. Be a child at play, no matter your age
10. Be a mover, not an exerciser
11. Be renewed by nature
12. Be insistent on rest
13. Be a stiff upper lipper
14. Be an optimistic ostrich
15. Be "one" and "we" above "I" and "me"
16. Be a jester, but know when to stay quiet
17. Be a servant
18. Be okay with being disliked
19. Be faithful to a higher Throne
20. Be kind to your face, and kindly face the inevitable
21. Be jubilant about aging
22. Be a jar of Marmite, always open to change
23. Be a bridge to the future

Source Notes

GOD SAVE MY GRACIOUS ME

As far as I can see [opening quote]: see Lacey, *The Crown*, 215.

"benign influence": "Why Do We Still Have a Monarchy?" a lecture presented by Jeremy Paxman, King's College London, June 27, 2008.

"a Sex Pistols attitude": Mirren, 220.

"magnified images": quoted in Longford, 173.

"the Queen has come to be": quoted in Bradford, 211.

"majesty of the ordinary": Lacey, *Majesty*, 7.

"When some of them did badly" [footnote]: Shawcross, *The Queen Mother*, 888.

Newspapers in London . . . again in the 1980s: see Longford, 173, 321–322.

"There is something about": Ibid.

"I would put some money": quoted in "The Queen's Subjects" by Boys of William Penn School in *Various*, 185–186.

"White Magic": quoted in Paxman, *On Royalty*, 125.

Readers of *The Lord of the Rings* [footnote]: see Day, 37; Tolkien, 871.

he laid hands on more than: see Starkey, 360.

"a great battle is lost": quoted in Smith, *Elizabeth the Queen*, xv.

"In her is incarnate": quoted in Paxman, *On Royalty*, 127.

"singularly blessed": Brown, *Ninety-Nine Glimpses*, 334.

"You can do a lot": quoted in Dolby, 23.

"a living archive": Bennett, 102.

"token of a better age": see Hughes, 112.

"She has served": "Elizabeth the Last" by Jonathan Freedland, *Guardian*, April 21, 2006.

"take all of her experiences": quoted in Andersen, *Game of Crowns*, 271.

"in the way wherein": quoted in Ratcliff, 48.

"You will therefore assume": *Cleopatra*, directed by Joseph Mankiewicz (Los Angeles, CA: 20th Century Fox, 1963).

"Out of nowhere": Mirren, 221, 229.

"I want to show": "Christmas Broadcast 1953," Royal Household website; royal.
uk, December 25, 1953.

"Papa. . . Gracious Me": quoted in Brown, *Ninety-Nine Glimpses*, 88.

"We is off" [footnote]: Dahl, 132.

EAT LIKE A QUEEN: OVERVIEW

Sometimes it is worth explaining [opening quote]: see Hamilton, 55.

"You will not photograph": quoted in Morrow, 112.

The solemn rites of royal: see Seward, *My Husband and I*, 242; Burgess, 244.

"Even if you are not finished": quoted in "10 Eating Habits of the Queen Revealed
by Royal Chef" by Kortney Gruenwald, Recipe Plus, accessed May 4, 2020.,

"if you indulged thoroughly": Blair, 150.

"the strange coupling": "What the Royals Eat at Home" by Rachel Cooke,
Guardian, May 19, 2012.

"Food is such an important": quoted in Shawcross, *Counting One's Blessings*, 380.

THE TUPPERWARE LADY

Middle-class "foodies" [opening quote]: Fox, 435–436.

"She is not particular": Smith, *Elizabeth the Queen*, 73.

"That sort of meal": John Gibson quoted in Bradford, 149.

"She sent a note": quoted in "10 Eating Habits of the Queen Revealed by Royal
Chef" by Kortney Gruenwald, Recipe Plus, accessed May 4, 2020.

They arrive "expecting banquets": Paxman, *On Royalty*, 5.

"not five-star enough": quoted in Paxman, *On Royalty*, 269.

"People don't come here": quoted in Hoey, *Life With the Queen*, 62.

"Cooking for [her]": quoted in Oliver, 192.

The Queen will not eat [footnote]: see Morrow, 108; James Whitaker quoted in
Secrets of the Royal Kitchen, directed by Andrew Sheldon, Timeline Documentaries, April 1, 2019.

"I have no intention" [footnote]: quoted in "Princess Margaret Dies at 71; Sister
of Queen Elizabeth Had a Troubled Life" by Joseph R. Gregory, *New York
Times*, February 10, 2002.

"I found this in my salad": quoted in Oliver, 20.

"complicated eaters": Shawcross, *Counting One's Blessings*, 585.

"a big round ball": quoting Tsar Nicholas II in Worsley, *Queen Victoria*, 324.

Near the front door: Paxman, *On Royalty*, 4.

"I didn't know what to do": Prince Charles quoted in Reagan, 16; referenced in Lyall, 117.

"dimensions and texture": see Andersen, *Game of Crowns*, 36.

he refuses to eat the local: see *Secrets of the Royal Kitchen,* directed by Andrew Sheldon, Timeline Documentaries, April 1, 2019.

It's said she took pleasure: see Bradford, 146.

Nanny Lightbody refused [footnote]: "Royal Nannies, Past and Present" by Kathryn Hughes, *Telegraph*, July 19, 2014.

The Queen Mother was raised: see Erickson, *Lilibet*, 27.

"hoosh-mi": see Crawford, 33.

To this day, whenever Elizabeth: see Smith, *Elizabeth the Queen*, 73.

4 oz. of sugar: see Williams, *Young Elizabeth*, 155.

The King insisted [footnote]: see Erickson, *Lilibet*, 67; Marr, 80.

chewed carrots . . . dropped an egg: see "Snoek Piquante" by Susan Cooper in Sissons, 35.

Longmate, 145.

Many historians agree: see Brown, *The Ration Book Diet*, 5; *Wartime Farm*, directed by Stuart Elliot, BBC Two, September 6, 2012.

"With every smell": quoted in Petrella, 80.

Mischel noticed that children: Mischel, 34–35, 134.

More recent studies: Ibid., 134.

Research shows that merely thinking [footnote]: see Logue, 14–15.

Top-drawer Brits: see Lyall; Fox; Paxman, *The English*.

"not being heated": Visser, 70.

"What's for lunch . . . Patience pudding": see in Casson, 7.

"wicker baskets, smoked salmon": Lyall, 1–2.

Hors d'oeuvres . . . bowl of crisps: see Smith, *Elizabeth the Queen*, 512.

"NEVER criticize the King or Queen": *Instructions for American Servicemen in Britain*, (Washington, DC: United States War Department, 1942); referenced in Williams, *Young Elizabeth*, 179.

QUEEN OF SCONES

One of the secrets [opening quote]: Murdoch, *The Sea*, 9.

400 feet of the daintiest: see Smith, *Elizabeth the Queen*, 173.

Prince Philip helped Elizabeth lose: Ibid., 54.

"Square Coffin": see Worsley, *Chocolate Fit for a Queen*, 10.

A little family ritual: see Crawford, 20.

"In our family": quoted in Morrow, 211.

Sitting beside a lace-lined cart . . . single leaf to escape: see Smith, *Elizabeth the Queen*, 73; Erickson, *Lilibet*, 227–228.

The flying-cake incident [footnote]: Erickson, *Lilibet*, 234.

"an exercise in grounding": Ibid., 225.

Afternoon visits with the Queen: see Hoey, *Life with the Queen*, 90.

A dedicated tea trunk: see Morrow, 118.

The first and most famous [footnote]: see Duhigg, 132–135.

"There's been more than two hundred": quoted in Duhigg, 135.

In studies where people: see Baumeister, 46–48.

"No glucose, no willpower": Ibid., 48.

"by sheer strength of willpower": quoted in Paterson, *A Brief History*, 8.

"jam pennies": see Andersen, *Game of Crowns*, 58.

"Beneath simple roofs": George Gissing, *The Private Papers of Henry Ryecroft*, quoted in Ingrams, 136.

The Victorian public: see Paxman, *On Royalty*, 100.

Elizabeth feels so much at home: see Morrow, 127.

"Life without fika": Brones, 1.

"positive procrastination": Baumeister, 234–235.

"even though every delicacy": Hoey, *Life with the Queen*, 90.

the groom's cake [footnote]: see "Queen Elizabeth II's Favorite Cake: Chocolate Biscuit Cake" by Darren McGrady, *Today*, April 4, 2017.

"The Queen is such . . . whole of that cake": see "Royal Chef Reveals Queen Elizabeth's Fave Meal and the One Thing She Hates," presented by Darren McGrady, *Delish*, January 15, 2020; quoted in "10 Eating Habits of the Queen Revealed by Royal Chef" by Kortney Gruenwald, Recipe Plus, accessed May 4, 2020.

Queen Victoria spent her childhood: Worsley, *Queen Victoria*, 47, 113.

"the craziest things to lose": York, 10.

"If we consciously deny": Wansink, 27.

"you must *not* be in too much": Crawford, 119.

TIARAS IF POSSIBLE

Table manners, which constitute [opening quote]: Visser, 73.

"I could eat all that!": quoted in Smith, *Diana in Search*, 171.

the quick fix of bulimia: Ibid., 110-111.

ancient term "courtesy": see Visser, 58.

Queen Mary . . . refused to touch: see Crawford, 258; Shawcross, *The Queen Mother*, 188.

"tiaras if possible": quoted in Longford, 16.

"Mach 2": quoted in Petrella, 80.

"small is beautiful": Fox, 443–444.

"I didn't know you didn't eat": Claire Foy in discussion with Chelsea Handler in "The Crown's Claire Foy," *Chelsea*, Netflix, December 7, 2017.

One works gracefully through the roll: see Morgan, *Debrett's New Guide*, 326.

This care also extends to tea [footnote]: "Royal Butler Reveals the Queen's Favorite Tea—and Whether She Pours the Milk in First" by Chloe Best, *Hello!*, April 26, 2019.

As a proponent of the politer: see Oliver, 51.

Since forks, when held upright: see Visser, 193.

"Denying a modern fork": Ibid.

"Life can be so difficult" [footnote]: quoted in Morrow, 92.

"You can't be seen with beans": quoted in *Secrets of the Royal Kitchen*, directed by Andrew Sheldon, Timeline Documentaries, April 1, 2019.

"to crumble or reduce": Visser, 173.

anytime she eats a banana: see "10 Eating Habits of the Queen Revealed by Royal Chef" by Kortney Gruenwald, Recipe Plus, accessed May 4, 2020.

"small is beautiful": Fox, 443.

"consumption snobbery" [footnote]: Rubin, *Better than Before*, 141.

Wallis Simpson collided with royal: see Sebba, 143.

"I have never hated anything": quoted in Shawcross, *Counting One's Blessings*, 486–487.

"If she were being served steak": unnamed Palace official in discussion with Smith, *Elizabeth the Queen*, 73.

She also prefers to serve herself: see Seward, *My Husband and I*, 248.

"That's the etiquette": quoted in *Secrets of the Royal Kitchen*, Timeline Documentaries.

"throwaway society" . . . "Dog leads" [footnote]: Marr, 7; see Bradford, 356; Hughes, 10; quoted in Longford, 226.

No matter how much food: see Wansink, 175.

The French, by contrast [footnote]: Ibid., 53.

It takes twenty minutes: see Lewis, 146.

hara hachi bu: see Garcia, 14; Stalker, 76; Buettner, *The Blue Zones*, 83.

Explanations often focus [footnote]: see Garcia, 126; Buettner, *The Blue Zones*, 83–84.

"So out of consideration": quoted in Smith, *Elizabeth the Queen*, 101.

She thinks it sounds too "vulgar" [footnote]: Hoey, *Life with the Queen*, 24.

"I am the last bastion" [footnote]: quoted in Hardman, *Queen of the World*, 13.

THE WINDSOR WETS' CLUB

The answer, if you ask [opening quote]: see Hamilton, 155.

In a perk that often surprises: see Hoey, *Life with the Queen*, 78.

aqua vitae non aqua pura: see Shawcross, *The Queen Mother*, 338.

"I hear you like gin": quoted in Lyall, 74.

"drinking powers": see Shawcross, *The Queen Mother*, 248.

"Would someone please come": quoted in Dolby.

"Where's the Southern Comfort" [footnote]: quoted in "Ninety Gaffes in Ninety Years," *Independent*, May 28, 2011.

"She'd be pickled": quoted in "Royal Chef Sets Record Straight on what Queen Elizabeth Eats and Drinks" by Susan Scutti, CNN, August 3, 2017.

take a nip from the flask of brandy: see Smith, *Elizabeth the Queen*, 88.

"The Queen's eyes were brimming": quoted in Ibid., 385.

Elizabeth also rarely missed: Ibid., 452.

Places like Sardinia . . . "it may also be": Buettner, *The Blue Zones*, 181.

"She loved social drinking": Burgess, *Behind Palace Doors*, 12.

"It's one of my little treats": quoted in Hamilton, 46.

"was simply unimaginable": Rhodes, 173.

The Queen Mother was a "steady" drinker: Tinniswood, 336.

"Water is NOT water" [footnote]: quoted in Brown, *Ninety-Nine Glimpses*, 120.

"Now, now, Lilibet": quoted in "William and Kate are Common Property" by Michael White, *Guardian*, April 28, 2011.

"abstemious": see Bradford, 149, 502.

Observers recounted how footmen [footnote]: see Morton, *Wallis in Love*, 67–68.

Hence one glass of pink vermouth: see Morrow, 53.

little more than plain tonic: see Longford, 7.

"self-transcendent" drinker: see Strecher, 123.

France lists only slightly: "AA Meetings in France," Alcoholics Anonymous (Continental European Region), 2019.

"Now I really do need": quoted in Erickson, *Lilibet*, 314.

WORK LIKE A QUEEN: OVERVIEW

My castle, my rules [opening quote]: *The King's Speech*, directed by Tom Hooper (New York, NY: The Weinstein Company).

dustpan and brush for the holidays: see Williams, *Young Elizabeth*, 45.

"the hardest worker of us all": "Why the Queen at 90 Is the Hardest Worker of Us All" by Matthew Dennison, *Telegraph*, April 20, 2016.

500 royal engagements: see Erickson, *Lilibet*, 134.

At age 82: see Smith, *Elizabeth the Queen*, 485.

hosting some 50,000 people: see Dolby, 45.

three hours to complete: see "Queen Elizabeth II," a lecture presented by Professor Vernon Bogdanor, the Museum of London, May 16, 2017.breaks for only two days: see Smith, *Elizabeth the Queen*, 71.

the Queen is never off duty: see Paxman, *On Royalty*, 62.

"Playing at king is no sinecure": quoted in Tinniswood, 188.

Previously a heavy smoker himself [footnote]: see Eade, 175.

"He literally died for England": Alexander Hardinge quoted in Brandreth, 85.

"To be heir to the throne": quoted in Paxman, *On Royalty*, 60.

"Poor you": quoted in Longford, 69.

"Is there any one of the royal family": quoted in "Exclusive: Prince Harry on Chaos After Diana's Death and Why the World Needs 'the Magic' of the Royal Family" by Angela Levin, *Newsweek*, June 6, 2017.

"I only hope they will not kill": quoted in Airlie, 236.

"give myself heart and soul": "Christmas Broadcast 1953," Royal Household website; royal.uk, December 25, 1953.

"an apparently inexhaustible electric charge": quoted in Paxman, *On Royalty*, 199.

"The Queen doesn't expect" [footnote]: quoted in Andersen, *Game of Crowns*, 243.

"firm level gaze": see Longford, 370.

THE MOST EXCELLENT ORDER OF ORDER

This sense of order was [opening quote]: Crawford, 19.

every day like clockwork: see Bradford, 29, 95.

"apart from even the question": quoted in Crawford, 97.

she carefully folded the paper: see Smith, *Elizabeth the Queen*, 14.

sometimes jumping out of bed: see Crawford, 116.

little more than childish "fretwork": quoted in Erickson, *Lilibet*, 59.

Princess Margaret could always get: see Crawford, 116.

"every day of your life": quoted in Hamilton, 112.

the Queen found "strength in": Erickson, *Lilibet*, 134.

There's always been a wake-up cup: for an overview of the Queen's daily routine see Smith, 69–74.

"Almost every year": Marr, 306.

consult the "Court Circular": available at https://www.royal.uk/court-circular.

heraldic motto *Semper Eadem*: see Levin, 1.

the longest-continuous institution: "The Monarchy," a lecture presented by David Starkey, Cambridge University, November 19, 2005.

King James I (1566–1625) liked to demonstrate [footnote]: see Paxman, *On Royalty*, 142.

"Poor Britannia": quoted in Rhodes, 162.

It was a "lesson" the Duchess: Ferguson, *What I Know Now*, 29.

"the comfort of the expected": Ibid.

"She has been there": quoted in Hardman, *Queen of the World*, 15.

"a beacon of tradition and stability": quoted in Smith, *Prince Charles*, 377.

"To be that consistent for that long": Helen Mirren in discussion with Smith, *Elizabeth the Queen*, xiv.

acts of repetition are crucial: see Duhigg.

In a study of workers: see S. Ohly et al., "Routinization, Work characteristics and their relationships with creative and proactive behaviors," *Journal of Organizational Behavior* 27 (2006): 257–279; referenced in Pang, 88.

"step for step, every day": "Dilbert Creator had Found a Brilliant Way to Trick Himself into Creativity" by Scott Adams, *Business Insider*, March 24, 2015.

"I am so glad to know": quoted in Shawcross, *Counting One's Blessings*, 360.

a "serenely" religious quality: Starkey, 491.

a modified "rule of life": Pierlot, 10, 25.

The Queen's timetable can be [footnote]: Bradford, 174.

"Zeigarnik effect": see Baumeister, 83–84.

"a hundred new ones": Pierlot, 25.

Writing down specific plans: see Baumeister, 83–84.

people who write down goals: study conducted by Gail Matthews, Dominican University of California, 2008; referenced in Keller, 154.

Imagine a playground: Chesterton, *G. K. Chesterton*, 375.

"the liberty to bind myself": Chesterton, *The Collected Works*, 328.

"Cicero once wrote": Csikszentmihalyi, 179.

"I tend to lead a sort of idiotic": quoted in Smith, *Prince Charles*, 134.

"was like nailing jellies": quoted in Dimbleby, 358.

William flourished under the school's: see Gordon, 228.

"It's simple really. All babies": Ashford, 221.

reportedly the only person [footnote]: "Margaret (Bobo) MacDonald; Dresser, Confidante to Queen," *Los Angeles Times*, September 25, 1993.

THE BUCKINGHAM SYSTEM

Beware! You are entering [opening quote]: see "The Prince and the Planet" by Bob Colacello, *Vanity Fair*, October 6, 2010.

save Christmas and Easter: see Smith, *Elizabeth the Queen*, 71.

"I must go do my boxes": quoted in Smith, *Elizabeth the Queen*, 72.

bygone era "of quiet tranquility": Hoey, *Life with the Queen*, 18.

"If you'll forgive me": quoted in Brandreth, 245.

"My initial intuition . . . utterly mad": Burgess, 18–19.

"extraordinarily respectful of other people": Greene, 34.

a mark of genuine disrespect: Ibid.

"Less dressy!" [footnote]: quoted in Leibovitz, 189.

"Imagine the Statue of Liberty's" [footnote]: Conrad, 73–74.

"Everybody I meet I vow". quoted by Peter Hennessy during Q&A of "Why Do We Still Have a Monarchy?" a lecture presented by Jeremy Paxman, King's College London, June 27, 2008.

"the Music Room": see "The Queen Spares Chirac His Waterloo" by David Millward, *Telegraph*, November 16, 2004.

translating Western concepts: see Levine, *A Geography of Time*, 177–178.

Even casually referring to your coworker: see "5 Major Differences Between Japanese and American Workplaces" by Yasmin Sara Merchant, *Business Insider*, April 5, 2018.

"hostility and anger": Levine, *A Geography of Time*, 178.

karoshi, "death from overwork" [footnote]: "How the Japanese are Putting an End to Extreme Work Weeks" by Danielle Demetriou, BBC, January 17, 2020.

"What is it?": quoted in "Queen is 'Not Amused' by Berlusconi Gaffe" by Anita Singh, *Telegraph*, April 3, 2009.

Years ago, American ambassador: see Smith, *Hostage to Fortune*, 253; Erickson, *Lilibet*, 182.

"I must let the Lord Lieutenant know": quoted in Erickson, *Lilibet*, 182.

242 · SOURCE NOTES

"any crisis could be handled": Ibid.

"Operation Overlord": see Lacey, *Monarch*, 358.

She might juggle more job titles: see Morgan, *The Audience*, 9–10.

"at her desk she is a marvel": Longford, 161.

"intellectual brilliance": quoted in "Why the Queen at 90 Is the Hardest Worker of Us All" by Matthew Dennison, *Telegraph*, April 20, 2016.

our brains are downright delinquent: see Keller.

"It keeps me up late at night . . . Multitaskers were just lousy": quoted in "The Mediocre Multitasker" by Ruth Pennebaker, *New York Times*, August 30, 2009.

Researchers now estimate: Keller, 46–47.

"There is nothing more fatiguing": quoted in Pope-Hennessy, 423.

Prince Andrew technically gave: see "There's at Least 1 Thing Elizabeth Has in Her Purse That You Probably Do Too" by Johnni Macke, MSN, July 18, 2019.

Prankster Prince Harry [footnote]: Ibid.

"I miss seeing their eyes": quoted in Hardman, *Queen of the World*, 13.

just plain "weird": Ibid.

According to former Google: see Price, 30–31.

Americans check their phones: Deloitte, 2018 Global Mobile Consumer Survey: US Edition.

"modern modes of communication": Ferguson, *What I Know Now*, 60.

"Do answer it, dear": quoted in Marr, 284.

"I am an amazing woman!": quoted in Smith, *Elizabeth the Queen*, 360.

A small decision like turning [footnote]: see Price.

Airs And Graces

Poise is Power [opening quote]: Shinn, 76.

"She's a stiffener of backs": quoted in Erickson, *Lilibet*, 191.

"Her curtsey almost" [footnote]: quoted in "The Real Elizabeth II: Part Two" by Graham Turner, *Telegraph*, January 9, 2002.

"Anna Anderson" [footnote]: see Paxman, *On Royalty*, 66.

"All the film people in the world": quoted in Williams, *Young Elizabeth*, 270.

"carriage of her head": Ibid., 184.

"What winning graces!": Pope, 78.

"in all her seventy-seven years": Seward, *The Queen's Speech*, 192.

"straight back . . . never slumped": quoted in Smith, *Elizabeth the Queen*, 111.

"a lady's back should never touch": Ibid., 13.

workers in any other industry sector: see Starrett, 7; E. Jensen, "Moving with the Brain in Mind," *Educational Leadership* 58 (2000): 34–37.

"There was no such thing as backache": Longford, 161.

"sit up at a slight distance": quoted in Smith, *Elizabeth the Queen*, 13.

Lee Albert recommends [footnote]: see *3 Steps to Pain Free Living* presented by Lee Albert, Inky Dinky Worldwide, Inc, 2019.

There's an iconic photograph: see Erickson, *Lilibet*, 55.

"magnificent carriage": Crawford, 22.

"Teach that child": quoted in Seward, *The Queen's Speech*, 20.

In a 1932 snapshot: see Crawford, inserted family photographs.

"bolt upright": Shawcross, *Counting One's Blessings*, 433.

All healthy babies do: see Porter; Starrett, 13, 16.

corrective shoulder pad [footnote]: see Hughes, 11.

"One plants one's feet": quoted in Bradford, 376.

The Queen instantly regained balance: referenced in Smith, *Prince Charles*, 498.

Elizabeth "will not entertain" [footnote]: Hughes, 14.

"an equanimity of body": Spark, 50.

Hormones like testosterone: see "Your Body Language May Shape Who You Are," a TED Talk presented by Amy Cuddy, June 2012; Peterson, 14–15, 26–28.

recovering alcoholics: D. Randles and J. L. Tracy, "Nonverbal Displays of Shame Predict Relapse and Declining Health in Recovering Alcoholics," *Clinical Psychological Science* (2013): 149–155.

struggle with depression . . . low energy: S. Nair, "Do Slumped and Upright Postures Affect Stress Responses? A Randomized Trial," *Health Psychology* 34 (2015): 632–641; L. Huang et al., "Powerful Postures versus Powerful Roles: Which Is the Proximate Correlate of Thought and Behavior?" *Psychological Science* 22 (2011): 95–102; E. Peper and I. Lin, "Increase or Decrease Depression: How Body Postures Influence Your Energy Level," *Biofeedback* 40 (2012): 125–130.

"a psychological cascade . . . a positive cycle": quoted in "The Right Stance Can Be Reassuring" by Kate Murphy, May 3, 2013.

In a 1999 study [footnote]: see Baumeister, 130–131.

"Your posture can define": Lubomirski, 59, 77.

"bigger, prouder, bolder": "The Queen: Majesty and Modesty" by John Walsh, *Independent*,

February 4, 2012.

the seven-page document: see Hoey, *Not in Front of the Corgis*, 18.

"Subjects seldom sulked": Bennett, 104.

VIVE LE DEVOIR

I will remain on the throne [opening quote]: see "Queen Margrethe Will Not Abdicate Anytime Soon" by Gabriel Aquino, *Royal Central*, February 26, 2018.

"Oh, that's something": quoted in Smith, *Elizabeth the Queen*, 515.

Monarchs throughout Europe: see "Duty Is the Key to the Queen's Success" by Lucy Draper, *Newsweek*, June 19, 2015.

"We have beheaded monarchs": unnamed senior courtier quoted in Morrow, 245.

"In this existence": quoted in "Why the Queen at 90 Is the Hardest Worker of Us All" by Matthew Dennison, *Telegraph*, April 20, 2016.

Elizabeth belongs to a generation: see Marr, 319.

"Wilhelmina is only sixty-eight": quoted in Pope-Hennessy, 576.

It's long been observed: see Buettner, *The Blue Zones*, 87.

Retirees soon experience: Gabriel H. Sahlgren, "Work Longer, Live Healthier," *Institute of Economic Affairs*, May 2013.

a life completely devoid of meaningful work: see Pang.

The long-lived Japanese: see Garcia.

If you enjoy your job [footnote]: see Friedman.

"the happiness of always being busy": Garcia, 2.

"I'm ninety-one": quoted in Smith, *Prince Charles*, 506–507.

If any member of the family: see Seward, *My Husband and I*, 181.

"It's no good sitting back": quoted in Shawcross, *Counting One's Blessings*, 868.

concept of eudaimonia: see Robertson, 8, 59.

"something special, a young king": Lee, 48.

"this feeling of being set aside": quoted in Seward, *My Husband and I*, 94.

"Everyone has his own": Frankl, 113.

has been shown to increase: see Strecher, 12–15.

In a now classic experiment: E. J. Langer and J. Rodin, "The Effects of Choice and Enhanced Personal Responsibility for the Aged: A Field Experiment in an Institutional Setting," *Journal of Personality and Social Psychology* 34 (1976): 191–198; referenced in Greenstein, 77–78.

"A slight flush on her face": quoted in Bradford, 166.

required sedatives: see Erickson, *Lilibet*, 132.

"When you're 'in purpose'": quoted in Santi, 38.

"no longer [felt] anxious": quoted in Williams, *Young Elizabeth*, 271.

"He who has a why": quoted in Frankl, 84.

"a bloody amoeba": quoted in Eade, 260.

a severe case of jaundice: Ibid., 264; Erickson, *Lilibet*, 158.

"depression can result" [footnote]: Santi, 42.

cleaning her seashell collection: see Brown, *Ninety-Nine Glimpses*, 269.

"She has no direction": quoted in ibid., 157.

"No one would talk to you": quoted in Bradford, 313.

"the absence of a role": Hugo Vickers quoted in Brown, *Ninety-Nine Glimpses*, 289.

"I have always had a dread": quoted in Petrella, 153.

"It is very simple": "A speech by the Queen on Her 21st Birthday," Royal House-hold website; royal.uk, April 21, 1947.

So important is this simple phrase: see Arbiter, 251.

"unique and alone in the universe": Frankl, 86.

starting comparisons [footnote]: see Strecher, 37.

"I didn't suddenly wake up": quoted in Seward, *My Husband and I*, 119; "Britain's Prince Charles: The Apprentice King," *Time*, June 27, 1969.

People who are driven: see Strecher, 29; Santi, 25.

"There was a shared philosophy": Anthony Clare in conversation with Brandreth, 115.

"This is the true joy": quoted in Strecher, 76.

"Remember that good spreads outward": quoted in Greene, 45.

"A big stone can cause waves": quoted in Seward, *The Queen's Speech*, 106.

"continuity" is the single [footnote]: see Marr, 9.

PLAY LIKE A QUEEN: OVERVIEW

I'm afraid Her Majesty [opening quote]: Bennett, 42.

In the summer of 1998: see Junor, *Prince William*, 148.

"It's not every day": quoted in "Harry's Climbing Caper 'Foolhardy,'" BBC News, August 9, 1998.

Fondly known as "Tiggy" [footnote]: see Junor, *Prince Harry*, 101.

"If I have done anything" [footnote]: quoted in Lear, 309.

"a healthy sense of fun": quoted in Smith, *Elizabeth the Queen*, 38.

They are *always* proven wrong: see Marr, 92.

"flash of colour": quoted in Lacey, *Monarch*, 159.

HER MAJESTY'S PLEASURE

It made him remember [opening quote]: White, 47.

"Oh, Crawfie": quoted in Crawford, 62.

"The last thing anyone": Ibid.

"catching the days": Margaret Rhodes in conversation with Smith, *Elizabeth the Queen*, 4.

joined their parents: see Crawford, 45.

production of Aladdin: see Pimlott, 77.

few children are able: see Brannen, 37.

"positively girlish": Judi James quoted in "Duchess of Sussex Brings Out Queen's Inner-Child: Body Language Expert Analyses Their First Joint Trip" by Gareth Davies and Hannah Furness, *Telegraph*, June 14, 2018.

"grey and grim": quoted in Smith, *Elizabeth the Queen*, 275.

"Wheeeeee!": Ibid., 274.

"Don't be silly!" Ibid., in discussion with Nancy Reagan, 320.

"catching out the minister": see Longford, 185.

"What did you think": quoted in Smith, *Elizabeth the Queen*, 93.

neoteny: see Brown, *Play*, 55.

"forever young": Ibid., 56–57.

crossover studies in humans: Ibid., 70–71.

"Merry Mischief": see Dolby, 89.

"I love life": quoted in Burgess, 171.

"naughty" escapades: Ibid.

"play history": Brown, *Play*.

"utterly irresistible mischievousness": quoted in Smith, *Prince Charles*, 374.

cheating at card games: see Marr, 56.

Lady Strathmore admired [footnote]: see Gordon, 199.

"We cavorted endlessly": Marr, 307.

"busy driving her team": quoted in Williams, *Young Elizabeth*, 62.

"I mostly go once or twice": Ibid., 62.

Crawfie was soon prancing: see Longford, 53.

riding her Fell ponies: see Smith, *Elizabeth the Queen*, 451.

flatulates and eats hay: the exact quote runs, "If it doesn't fart or eat hay, she isn't interested"; "Wince Philip: Philip's Most Famous Comments and Clangers," *Guardian*, May 4, 2017.

"the one subject": Michael Oswald quoted in Shawcross, *Queen and Country*, 182.

"heart play": see Brannen, xiii.

"your heart sing": Ibid., xiii.

"a turning point in my fate": Carl Jung quoted in Dunne, 67.

known as "flow": see Csikszentmihalyi.

"deep play": see Pang, 201.

"Play is more than just fun": title of TED Talk presented by Stuart Brown, Serious Play 2008.

"Her responsibilities as monarch": quoted in Shawcross, *Queen and Country*, 182.

"When the horses run well": quoted in Bradford, 256.

She had no discernable hobbies: see Smith, *Diana in Search*, 106.

"She was an empty vessel": Ibid., 106.

"the opposite of play": "Play Is More Than Just Fun," a TED Talk presented by Stuart Brown, 2008.

"she rehearsed court receptions": quoted in Worsley, *Queen Victoria*, 48.

"Riding taught [her]": Longford, 365.

"equine" therapy [footnote]: see Hayes; Ferguson, *Finding Sarah*, 184.

study out of North Dakota: D. L. Zabelina and M. D. Robinson, "Child's Play: Facilitating the Originality of Creative Output by a Priming Manipulation," *Psychology of Aesthetics, Creativity, and the Arts*, 4, no. 1 (2010): 57–65.

when children are given: "The Importance of Recess," *Harvard Health Publishing*, July 2015.

The first charity William: see Junor, *Prince William*, 357.

"You couldn't feel properly sad": Longford, 200.

Children turn to play: see Brannen, 28.

"Paradox of Control . . . where any number": Csikszentmihalyi, 59.

"into another dimension": quoted in Smith, *Prince Charles*, 154.

"Do you know there is one thing": quoted in Longford, 169.

FIT TO RULE

Horses sweat [opening quote]: see Casson, 14.

"Oh look!": quoted in Marr, 284.

"like a liner": Ibid., 248.

"I'm as strong": quoted in Smith, 82; Erickson, *Lilibet*, 207.

"My grandmother warned" [footnote]: quoted in Morrow, 78.

"When we sat down" [footnote]: quoted in Brandreth, 88.

endurance is "striking": Smith, *Elizabeth the Queen*, 278.

"You need not worry": Ibid., 278.

never sits at Palace events: see Hoey, *Life with the Queen*, 12.

"great assets": quoted in Smith, *Elizabeth the Queen*, xvii.

A little-known requirement: see Hoey, 124.

"left even the Secret Service": quoting in "A Royal Couple Receives A Presidential Welcome" by Karen de Witt, *New York Times*, May 15, 1991.

Insisting on wearing: see Erickson, *Lilibet*, 141, 219.

carrying two bags of sugar: see Hoey, *We Are Amused*, 171.

"your neck would break" [footnote]: Elizabeth II in discussion with Alastair Bruce, *The Coronation*, directed by Harvey Lilley, BCC One, May 27, 2008.

Philip used to pile on: see Seward, *My Husband and I*, 77.

"dynamo" . . . "crackled with energy": quoting Mike Parker and Patricia Mountbatten in Brandreth, 198.

"I think Prince Philip is mad": quoted in Bradford, 147; "Great Britain: The Queen's Husband" *Time*, October 21, 1957.

"puffed," as she calls it: see Smith, *Elizabeth the Queen*, 182.

"is a great believer": Seward, *The Queen's Speech*, 203.

every day around two thirty: see Andersen, *Game of Crowns*, 58; Hoey, *We Are Amused*, 94.

"intentionally measured": quoted in Smith, *Elizabeth the Queen*, xiii.

"rarely used except by": Brown, *The Diana Chronicles*, 370.

On the Italian island: see Buettner, *The Blue Zones Solution*, 56.

"regular, low-intensity": Ibid., 56.

"You'll never see me": Dan Buettner quoted in "My Dinner with Longevity Expert Dan Buettner (No Kale Required)" by Jeff Gordinier, *New York Times*, April 1, 2015.

"She didn't have a bead" [footnote]: quoted in Smith, *Elizabeth the Queen*, 105.

"More is in you": see Williams, *Young Elizabeth*, 146.

The school day began: see Eade, 96.

"I should think as little": Ibid., 96.

"loved walking . . . young enough": Crawford, 4, 9.

They went on mile-long marches: see Erickson, *Lilibet*, 56.

"only mildly strenuous": Ibid., 56.

"Exercise is different": York, 13.

"Our movement intensity": Segar, 7.

1996 report from the US Surgeon: *Physical Activity and Health: A Report of the Surgeon General* (Atlanta: GA: US Department of Health and Human Services, 1996).

"But getting people": Segar, 72.

wonders of NEAT: see Levine.

"profoundly more powerful": James Levine quoted in "Keep on Moving" by Catherine Jarvie, *Guardian*, July 1, 2005.

"People who have the ability" [footnote]: Levine, *Get Up!*, 31.

"a major bit of exercise": Sarah Ferguson, *Finding Sarah*, 29.

"all far too big": Crawford, 85, 82.

a good five minutes: Ibid., 85.

"People here need bicycles": Ibid., 93.

"ventilation threshold": see Segar, 58–59; Panteleimon Ekkekakis et al., "The Pleasure and Displeasure People Feel When They Exercise at Different Intensities: Decennial Update and Progress towards a Tripartite Rationale for Exercise Intensity Prescription," *Sport Medicine* 41 (2011): 641–671.

On average, people drop [footnote]: Segar, 6, 19.

"an obsession for her": James Hewitt quoted in Smith, *Diana in Search*, 178.

more refreshed and renewed: see Seward, *The Queen's Speech*, 6.

66 percent more people: see "Volkswagen Brings the Fun: Giant Piano Stairs and Other 'Fun Theory' Marketing" by Kelsey Ramon, *Los Angeles Times*, October 15, 2009.

"Fun is the easiest way": Ibid.

Dog owners, for instance: see Rubin, *Better than Before*, 95.

"when we view it as a gift": Segar, 41.

"alone" time: see Andersen, *Game of Crowns*, 58.

"I have walked myself" [footnote]: see Marino, 39.

relaxation response [footnote]: see "Exercising to Relax," *Harvard Health Publishing*, July 13, 2018.

"the first two days" [footnote]: Junor, *Prince William*, 123.

"She drove her own": quoted in Smith, *Elizabeth the Queen*, 451.

TWEEDY MODE

When duty calls me [opening quote]: "Over the Hills and Far Away," traditional English folk song, modern lyrics by John Tams, recorded in *Over The Hills and Far Away: The Music of Sharpe*, 1996.

picking up dead birds: a reference to one of the Queen's favorite country pastimes—retrieving the fallen grouse (with the help of her dogs) during shooting parties at Balmoral and, occasionally, soundly dispatching it with a stick if the bird wasn't quite dead; see Smith, *Elizabeth the Queen*, 201.

Diana had no intention: see Smith, *Diana in Search*, 170.

"grown men trying to throw": quoted in Hoey, *Life with the Queen*, 59.

"Does the prime minister": quoted in Smith, *Elizabeth the Queen*, 292.

"The Queen and I": Sarah Ferguson quoted in Smith, *Diana in Search*, 170.

"I love to get my hands": quoted in "Royal Duties? I'd Rather be Gardening Confesses Camilla" by Richard Palmer, *Sunday Express*, June 22, 2018.

heal the rift in 2000: see Andersen, *Game of Crowns*, 185.

"is clearly a country girl" [footnote]: quoted in Andersen, *William and Kate*, 138.

"The Queen is going" [footnote]: Ibid., 138.

"Until I came . . . rather grubby": Crawford, 29.

"Farmer George": see Flanagan, 30.

pulling up weeds in the garden: see Williams, *Young Elizabeth*, 55.

Wheeled outdoors while still in her pram: see Shawcross, *The Queen Mother*, 258.

"be as much in the open" [footnote]: quoted in Rappaport, 150.

"a lifelong passion" [footnote]: Worsley, *Queen Victoria*, 72.

positively "dissolved" [footnote]: Rappaport, 150.

"We were raised to believe": Rhodes, 38.

British nannies religiously: see Holden, 44, 162.

"Fresh air makes for healthy": see Ashford, 49.

"She is very strong": quoted in Crawford, 110.

"fond memories": quoted in Hampton, 284.

"I had a feeling" [footnote]: quoted in Smith, *Elizabeth the Queen*, 189.

"There is nothing like chopping": Ibid., 120.

"For a woman who is constantly": Seward, *The Queen's Speech*, 2.

Just pulling up a few weeds: see Erickson, *Lilibet*, 212.

"primal communion": Smith, *Elizabeth the Queen*, 204.

fishing in the frigid River Dee: see Shawcross, *The Queen Mother*, 799.

"fresh strength from the everlasting": quoted in Shawcross, *Counting One's Blessings*, 362.

"soft fascination" of nature: see Kaplan; Li, 110.

reduce our stress levels: Li, 176; "Fractal Patterns in Nature and Art are Aesthetically Pleasing and Stress-Reducing" by Richard Taylor, *The Conversation*, March 30, 2017.

"There is no medicine" [footnote]: Li, 109.

"always the fresh" [footnote]: Bradford, 74.

"languishing indoors": quoted in Smith, *Elizabeth the Queen*, 451.

"country house" weekend: Blair, 150.

"I do rather begrudge": quoted in Brandreth, 341.

"To lie sometimes on the grass": Lubbock, 69; referenced in Pang, 246.

All four of them developed a deep: see Smith, *Elizabeth the Queen*, 211–212.

ritually smeared with the blood: Ibid., 212.

"The natural habitat" [footnote]: Rhodes, 33.

every bit and bob [footnote]: see Burgess, 178.

"pure luxury . . . Scots pines": Princess Anne, 2, 16.

"The Old Man of Lochnager": see Smith, *Prince Charles*, 44.

he talks to his garden vegetables: see Petrella, 96; Hamilton, 99.

he would be a farmer: see Junor, *Prince William*, 53.

The "boys adored it": Ibid., 52.

Diana rarely joined them: Ibid., 54.

"I give them what they need": Alexandra Legge-Bourke quoted in Ibid., 81.

royal destiny repeating itself: see Smith, *Elizabeth the Queen*, 62.

Earl of Strathmore [footnote]: see Forbes, 7–9; Brandreth, 63.

"so well versed" [footnote]: Erickson, *Lilibet*, 33.

HIBERNATE

Labor is a craft [opening quote]: Heschel, 14.

"more dead than alive": quoted in Worsley, *Queen Victoria*, 232.

Diana took second place: see Smith, *Prince Charles*, 134; Junor, *Prince William*, 54.

"he never, ever stops thinking": Malcolm Ross, Charles's Master of the Household, quoted in Smith, *Prince Charles*, 416.

"He never, ever stops working" [footnote]: Ibid., 481.

"it's nice to hibernate": quoted in *Elizabeth R: A Year in the Life of the Queen*, directed by Edward Mirzoeff, BBC, February 6, 1992.

never had a genuine holiday: see Hoey, *Life with the Queen*, 55.

"tours" abroad have all been work-away trips: see Hardman, *Queen of the World*, 23.

"Sunbathing": Hoey, *Life with the Queen*, 55.

far more introverted: see Shawcross, *Queen and County*, 27.

"The world's most famous introvert": see "Why Queen Elizabeth Is the World's Most Famous Introvert" by Zahra Pettican, *Reader's Digest*, March, 2018.

introverts recharge very, very differently: see Cain, 10.

"as a goldfish in a bowl": quoted in "Never a Natural Second Fiddle" by Olga Craig, *Telegraph*, February 10, 2002.

Unlike her other country estate: see Smith, *Elizabeth the Queen*, 199.

"You can go out for miles": quoted in *Elizabeth R: A Year in the Life of the Queen*, directed by Edward Mirzoeff, BBC, February 6, 1992.

"Lights were going out": Crawford, 142.

"The very idea of a vacation" [footnote]: Hoey, *Life with the Queen*, 55.

As a girl she became restless [footnote]: see Crawford, 56.

"deliberate rest" [footnote]: see Pang, 14–15.

"hobbies that demand skill" [footnote]: Csikszentmihalyi, 162.

Charles Darwin . . . Dr. Seuss: see Cain, 83, 86.

"Solitude matters": see "The Power of Introverts," a TED Talk presented by Susan Cain, February 2012.

"homeliness" of the yacht: unnamed politician quoted in Marr, 162.

other monarchies . . . royal yachts: see Shawcross, *Queen and Country*, 205.

Churchill got into the habit: see Pang, 111.

"one of the inflexible rules": quoted in Paterson, *Winston Churchill*, 28.

"Nature," he argued: Churchill, 375.

"She takes her holidays": Greene, 61.

THINK LIKE A QUEEN: OVERVIEW

When the odds are hopeless [opening quote]: Fleming, 14.

"Good evening, Mr. Bond": from the short film, *Happy and Glorious* directed by Danny Boyle for the 2012 Summer Olympics Opening Ceremony, July 27, 2012.

"Go, Granny!": quoted in "London 2012 Olympics: Prince's Delight at Bond Girl Queen" by Andrew Hough, *Telegraph*, October 30, 2012.

"She is the most reliable": Seward, *The Queen's Speech*, 2.

"She has uttered": Marr, 69.

shot at . . . cricket ball: see Smith, *Elizabeth the Queen*, 188, 300, 301, 315; Erickson, *Lilibet*, 244.

"I never saw her scared": quoted in Smith, *Elizabeth the Queen*, 301.

"She didn't scream": Dahl, 151.

"never having to look": quoted in Smith, *Elizabeth the Queen*, xvii.

"the sweetest air": Anne Ring quoted in Erickson, *Lilibet*, 16.

"to get calmer": quoted in Smith, *Elizabeth the Queen*, 188.

"We're like sort of ducks": quoted in Petrella, 8.

THE MERRY STOICS OF WINDSOR

The duty which has befallen you [opening quote]: Morgan, *The Audience*, 13.

"people's princess": "Blair Pays Tribute to Diana," BBC News, September 1, 1997.

"a giant step closer": "Express Opinion: The Queen Must Lead Us in Our Grief," *Daily Express*, September 4, 1997; referenced in Dixon, 303.

"Show Us You Care": quoted in "The Queen Bows to Her Subjects" by Michael Streeter, *Independent*, September 5, 1997.

"inestimable services": Winston Churchill's address to the House of Commons on the occasion of Prince Charles's birth, November 16, 1948, accessed May 4, 2020, https://api.parliament.uk/historic-hansard/commons/1948/nov/16/birth-of-a-prince-address-of

Margaret Thatcher every week: see Greene, 32.

Suez crisis of 1956: see Waller, 6.

"courage to be boring": quoted in Hardman, *Queen of the World*, 11.

"never complain, never explain": see Burgess, 81.

"utterly discreet" [footnote]: Junor, *Prince William*, 360.

she was "brought up": quoted in Smith, *Elizabeth the Queen*, 13.

"make a fuss": a frequent observation of her governess, Marion Crawford; see Crawford.

"I've been trained since childhood": quoted in Seward, *My Husband and I*, 42.

"Hanoverian spleen": see Williams, *Young Elizabeth*, 16.

name of "gnashes": see Smith, *Elizabeth the Queen*, 6.

"He was not an easy man": quoted in Brandreth, 67.

Expensive furnishings: see Bradford, 519.

"I'd like to shoot them all!" [footnote]: quoted in Williams, *Young Elizabeth*, 203.

part his hair . . . porcelain sink: "Bedtime Stories" by Michelle Green, *People*, January 30, 1995.

"left hook": quoted in Erickson, *Lilibet*, 29.

"goaded by boredom": Crawford, 22.

her mother's calm and soothing example: see Smith, *Elizabeth the Queen*, 13.

"To wave, not to cry": quoted in Seward, *My Husband and I*, 43.

a roughly hundred-year period: see Dixon, 3–4.

"the noble generation": quoted in Marr, 270.

"people were held responsible": Csikszentmihalyi, 23.

"It was a different world": quoted in Brandreth, 78.

"narcissism and intolerance": quoted in Lyall, 232.

"mustn't grumble": see Paxman, *The English*, 1.

"Rather than taking it" [footnote]: Lyall, 236.

"The stiff upper lip": Brandreth, 92.

Stoicism the philosophy: see Pigliucci; Robertson.

"a zombie-like state": Irvine, 38.

"real strength lies in the *control*": Holiday, *The Obstacle Is the Way*, 30.

British psychologists feared: see Furedi, 217.

"Never Flinch, Never Weary": quoted in Burgess, 112.

"get on with it": see Lyall, 243.

BBC Broadcaster: see "Bruce and the Bomb" by Robert Seatter, BBC, October 14, 2010.

Aberfan disaster: see Furedi, 19.

"The villagers had done admirably": Ibid., 19.

"victimhood culture" [footnote]: see Lukianoff, 209.

The only time the Queen: see Greene, 55–56; Burgess, 30.

"Few of us are likely": Greene, 55–56.

"1992 is not a year": see "A Speech by the Queen on the 40th Anniversary of Her Accession (Annus Horribilis Speech)," Royal Household website; royal.uk, November 24, 1992.

"from the heart, not the head": Princess Diana's *Panorama* interview with Martin Bashir, BBC, November 20, 1995.

"preferred talking to repressing": Lyall, 232.

embarrassed William: see Junor, *Prince William*, 130–131.

"He's taken a leaf": Ibid., 309.

"a steady bloke": Ibid., 324.

"I think he has an innate sense": Ibid., 4.

"psychological armour": Ibid., 225.

"He's someone you'd like": Ibid., 4.

emotional "finesse": quoted in Edwards, 264.

nobilitas animi: "The Seed of Nobility," a lecture presented by Andrew Frisardi, Temenos Academy, Lincoln Centre, December 12, 2018.

"If" poem [footnote]: see "The Remarkable Story Behind Rudyard Kipling's "If"—and the Swashbuckling Renegade Who Inspired It" by Geoffrey Wansell, *Daily Mail*, February 15, 2009; Longford, 320.

most romantic movie [footnote]: see "*Brief Encounter* Is Named 'Most Romantic Movie' of All Time" by Hannah Furness, *Telegraph*, April 23, 2013.

"The Britons of this generation": "'We Will Meet Again'—the Queen's Coronavirus Broadcast," BBC, April 5, 2020.

50 percent of the public: see Mandler, 237.

what most people look back on: see Fox, 517–518.

OSTRICHING

Don't be defeatist [opening quote]: Fellowes, 51.

off bounds to a critical press: see Hamilton, 16.

"imperial ostrich": see Shawcross, *The Queen Mother*, 890.

"pursuit of happiness": Brown, *Ninety-Nine Glimpses*,125.

"groping in the darkness . . . misery": quoted in Shawcross, *The Queen Mother*, 381, 383.

"very depressed and miserable": Ibid., 375.

Like Victoria . . . weakness: see Worsley, *Queen Victoria*, 50.

acted like a "vampire": Shawcross, *Counting One's Blessings*, 412.

"I am still just as frightened": Ibid., 305.

"keep the old flag flying": Ibid., 171.

"the most dangerous woman": see Williams, *Young Elizabeth*, 190.

"so much easier to yell": quoted in Shawcross, *Counting One's Blessings*, 421.

"the happiness business": quoted in Paxman, *On Royalty*, 215.

"whatever is noble": Philippians 4:8, *Holy Bible*, New International Version.

"all the things I like . . . a million more": quoted in Shawcross, *Counting One's Blessings*, 127–128.

"least said soonest mended": see Brandreth, 314.

"Temperamentally she was": Longford, 21.

"this intolerable honour": quoted in Rhodes, 41.

"not once in all the years": Ibid., 41.

"Oh, they really are": quoted in Burgess, 74.

"The Queen Mother . . . reminded": Ibid., 73.

ostrich feathers [footnote]: Marr, 26.

"became adept at blocking": Ibid., 56.

"well, that was a fair-to-average": quoted in Morrow, 65.

"I find that I can often": quoted in Erickson, *Lilibet*, 200.

"When things are horrible": Burnett, 175.

"uninhibited emotional openness": Sommers, 7.

"For many temperaments": Ibid., 7.

"You just told . . . bankrupt" [footnote]: quoted in Ferguson, *Finding Sarah*, 96.

negativity drastically reduces: see Fredrickson, 164; S. Nolen-Hoeksema et al., "Rethinking Rumination," *Perspectives on Psychological Science* 3 (2008): 400–424.

"impose a lens . . . immobility": quoted in Sommers, 123–124.

sudden infant death . . . AIDS victims: Ibid., 136.

"some things are best not discussed": Burgess, 34.

when Prince Edward telephoned: see Seward, *The Queen's Speech*, 16.

Queen Mother liked to say, "unhelpful": see Brown, *Ninety-Nine Glimpses*, 125.

"purposeful repressor": see Sommers, 120.

Studies have shown . . . heart attack patients: Ibid., 120–121.

"The moods of repressed" [footnote]: J. Bybee et al., "Is Repression Adaptive? Relationships to Socioemotional Adjustment, Academic Performance, and Self-Image," *American Journal of Orthopsychiatry* 67 (1997): 59–69.

"We must learn not to hold": Plato; referenced in Furedi, 160.

Throughout the 1970s: see Seward, *The Queen's Speech*, 96.

"Perhaps we make . . . more depression": Ibid., 104.

"the psychological equivalent": Irvine, 218.

"throwing it up an imaginary": quoting Andrew Morton in Smith, *Diana in Search*, 188.

It's been recognized [footnote]: see Sommers, 112; R. Hornberger, "The Differential Reduction of Aggressive Responses as a Function of Interpolated Activities," *American Psychology* 14 (1959): 354.

"take all the aggro": quoted in Smith, *Diana in Search*, 188.

"as unsure of herself": Ibid., 362.

"I found in the end . . . squash you back": Ibid., 332.

"emotional hemophilia": Ibid., 366.

push tissues under the bathroom: see Morton, *Diana*, 276.

focus on "something positive": see Smith, *Diana in Search*, 275.

"Resilient people . . . harming me?": "The Three Secrets of Resilient People," a TED Talk presented by Lucy Hone, August 2019.

"free your mind and your bottom": quoted on back cover of Ferguson, *Finding Sarah*.

"negative mind chatter . . . poop balloons": Ibid., 284.

"powerful sadness . . . about 700" [footnote]: Gilbert, 137, 178.

VIEW FROM ABOVE

She must be above everything [opening quote]: Shawcross, *Counting One's Blessings*, 229.

array of national newspapers: see Brandreth, 207.

'it took up too much time' [footnote]: Shawcross, *Queen and County*, 162.

"I don't read the tabloids": quoted in Andersen, *Game of Crowns*, 44.

Time put her . . . afternoon walks: see Erickson, *Lilibet*, 23.

"adored . . . take it personally": Brandreth, 181.

"Good morning . . . hopes to be a lady": quoted in Seward, *My Husband and I*, 42.

"Oh, you can't . . . pay anything": quoted in Crawford, 192.

"Here we have the most": "Duty Is the Key to the Queen's Success" by Lucy Draper, *Newsweek*, June 19, 2015.

least desire to watch "herself": see Smith, *Elizabeth the Queen*, 466.

"She cares not for celebrity": "Duty Is the Key," *Newsweek*.

"I really don't know!" [footnote]: quoted in Shawcross, *The Queen Mother*, 167.

"Oh, please don't worry" [footnote]: quoted in "A Right Royal Mess Up!" by Roya Nikkhah, *Telegraph*, November 11, 2012.

"She sounds much too grand": quoted in Morrow, 2.

"corroding . . . not to do that": quoted in Brandreth, 181.

Diana troubled Elizabeth: Ibid., 321.

"Oh! This is the life": quoted in Smith, *Diana in Search*, 81.

"fallen in love with an idea": quoting Penny Romsey in Ibid., 95.

analyzing every story written: Ibid., 16.

"Diana got pulled . . . bothered her": Ibid., 16, 146.

"I didn't like , , , perform": Ibid., 16.

"the longer you look": Conrad, 103.

"I love myself more": Ferguson, *Finding Sarah*, 190–191.

few realize . . . Maslow changed his mind": see Strecher, 63.

"The fully developed": Ibid., 63.

"transcenders": Ibid., 63.

"lesson of modesty . . . human good": Marr, 319.

"opposite of Diana . . . talk about herself": unnamed courtier quoted in Smith, *Diana in Search*, 123.

"We are not amused" [footnote]: Hamilton, 28.

"We are a grandmother" [footnote]: quoted in "Margaret Thatcher: First Among Unequals" by Andy McSmith, *Independent*, June 30, 2010.

"They [prime ministers] know": quoted in Shawcross, *Queen and County*, 70.

"View from Above": Hadot; referenced in Robertson, 216–217.

"light above politics" [footnote]: quoted in Scruton, 188.

servants as footstools [footnote]: see Jaques, lxv.

"Survey the circling stars": Aurelius, 112.

"placid detachment . . . virtually everything": quoting in Burgess, 29, 80.

"overwhelming feelings . . . fly on the wall": E. Kross et al., "When Asking 'Why' Does Not Hurt: Distinguishing Rumination from Reflective Processing of Negative Emotions," *Psychological Science* 16 (2005): 709–715; referenced in Mischel, 150–151.

Subsequent studies: O. Ayduk and E. Kross, "Enhancing the Pace of Recovery: Self-Distanced Analysis of Negative Experiences Reduces Blood Pressure Reactivity," *Psychological Science* 19 (2008): 229–231; O. Ayduk and E. Kross, "From a Distance: Implications of Spontaneous Self-Distancing for Adaptive Self-Reflection," *Journal of Personality and Social Psychology* 98 (2010): 809–829; referenced in Mischel, 151–152.

"not revelations of absolute" [footnote]: Mischel, 153.

"evil Camilla" . . . "most hated woman": see "Camilla at 70: Has the Duchess Finally Won British Hearts?" by Kiko Itasaka, *NBC*, July 16, 2017.

"I was always brought up": quoted in Smith, *Prince Charles*, 333.

"Rottweiler . . . double chins": Ibid., 314.

"likened to Miss Piggy": Marr, xi.

"Oh Philip, do look!": Smith, *Elizabeth the Queen*, 303.

"Happiness is a matter": Murdoch, *The Nice*, 180–181; quoted in Brandreth, 330.

STINKING WILLIE

Oh look, Margo's on fire! [opening quote]: see Burgess, 154.

"to wipe his nether end": quoting Sir Thomas Heneage in Weir, *Henry VIII*, 81.

Stinking Willie . . . noxious weed": see Smith, *Elizabeth the Queen*, xvi.

"the Crown . . . does get rather heavy": quoted in Strong, 122.

Office of the Revels: see Greenstein, 89.

"a leap, a whistle": see Visser, 105.

"cured her melancholy": quoting Thomas Fuller in Tinniswood, 72.

chain of beacons to be lit: see "100 Bonfires Mark Elizabeth's Jubilee" by R. W. Apple Jr., *New York Times*, June 7, 1977.

"Your majesty . . . what fun!": quoting Major Sir Michael Parker, "A Right Royal Mess-Up!" by Roya Nikkhah, *Telegraph*, November 11, 2012.

"the only thing that keeps": Hoey, *Life with the Queen*, 44.

"Laughter, and a lot": Seneca, 33.

"I will swear to anyone" [footnote]: quoted in Irvine, 147.

"It may sound silly" [footnote]: Lukianoff, 241.

"Have you got a prison record": quoted in Marr, 163.

performed a mock curtsey: see Eade, 198.

range of practical jokes: Brandreth, 209.

"dontopedalogy . . . foot in it": quoted in Eade, 282.

"What do you gargle . . . cowboys and Indians": quoted in Dolby, 26, 56; "Prince Philip's Gaffes from Decades on Royal Duty," BBC, May 4, 2017.

"Aren't most of you . . . your beard" [footnote]: quoted in Dolby, 71–72; "Prince Philip's Gaffes from Decades on Royal Duty," BBC, May 4, 2017.

"has done the state": quoted in Brandreth, 209.

"common sight at parties": Ibid., 209.

"extremely funny in private": quoted in Dolby, 7.

her Yorkshire accent: see Smith, *Elizabeth the Queen*, 315.

"It looks very damp . . . New Zealand eggs": quoted in Dolby, 67, 69.

"Please tell the band": quoted in Bradford, 230.

"You should have" [footnote]: quoted in Smith, *Elizabeth the Queen*, 471.

"I've seen the Queen laugh": quoted in Bradford, 260.

"like an angry thunder-cloud": Crossman, 43–44; referenced in Marr, 179.

"blackly furious": Ibid.

"You know, I nearly laughed": Ibid.

"When she looked terribly angry": Ibid.

"Elizabeth appears to have applied": see "The Queen's Self-Abnegation Is About Self-Interest, Not Just Duty" by Deborah Orr, *Guardian*, September 9, 2015.

"reticent . . . reasons for silence": Longford, 111.

"Queen Mary moved on . . . awkward situation" [footnote]: quoting Mabell, Countess of Airlie in Longford, 126.

"an expert semiotician": Conrad, 76.

"icy silence": Marr, 69.

"She never argues": Ibid., 182.

a crucial "talent": quoted in Shawcross, *Queen and County*, 190.

positively "purring": see Bradford, 226.

"feeling marvelously refreshed": Morrow, 156.

"on the psychiatrist's couch": quoted in Paxman, *On Royalty*, 175.

people generally emerge from: see Marr, 11.

"If this is a strangely passive": Ibid., 319.

"considered inaction": quoted in Bradford, 485.

"Probably in most cases": Bagehot, 71.

"bear and forbear" [footnote]: quoted in Holiday, *The Obstacle Is the Way*, 131.

"Remember the two nice" [footnote]: quoted in Casson, 43.

"Sometimes we need . . . the enemy" [footnote]: Holiday, *The Obstacle Is the Way*, 110–111.

"If you are in a position of leadership": Salmon.

LOVE LIKE A QUEEN: OVERVIEW

My crown is in my heart [opening quote]: Shakespeare, *Henry VI*, 51.

one-third of all Britons: see Andersen, *Game of Crowns*, 1.

the commonalities are marvelous: see Paxman, *On Royalty*, 9–10.

"a really nice woman": quoted in Erickson, *Royal Panoply*, 324.

wasn't "huggy" enough: see Marr, 270.

"If only [Meghan] could" [footnote]: "Why Does Meghan Markle Need to Be So Huggy Wuggy?" by Jan Moir, *Daily Mail*, February 15, 2018.

pocket money . . . ballet slippers: see Seward, *The Queen's Speech*, 26.

mothers of fallen soldiers: see Crawford, 195.

"For a child of her years": Williams, *Young Elizabeth*, 210.

"Mama belong big family": see "Papua New Guinea," Royal Household website; royal.uk.

NOBLESSE OBLIGE

There is a motto [opening quote]: see Seward, *The Queen's Speech*, 32.

more of his own wealth: see Paxman, *On Royalty*, 138–139.

King Farouk of Egypt predicted: Ibid., 7.

"best defined as the power": Pope-Hennessy, 427.

90 charitable . . . 3,500 under Elizabeth: see Shawcross, *Queen and Country*, 96.

"charitable bulldozer": quoted in Marr, 32.

three to four hospital visits: see Paxman, *On Royalty*, 225.

"I'm tired and I hate hospitals": Ibid., 225.

"an astonishing gift . . . enjoy it" [footnote]: Ibid., 229.

Ich Dien, "I serve": see Tinniswood, 292.

"Can't you understand . . . brief reign": Ibid., 292.

"assured him . . . note to the gardener": Crawford, 175.

"It is my resolve": quoted in Longford, 181.

visit a leper colony: see "The Role Elizabeth Was Born to Play" by Amanda Foreman, *Telegraph*, February 12, 2012.

number of charities: see "The Queen's Birthday: How She Became Patron of 600 Organisations," BBC News, June 12, 2016; "The Queen Has Done More for Charity than Any Other Monarch in History" by Kate Hodge, *Guardian*, June 11, 2012.

"the Queen has done": "The Queen Has Done," *Guardian*.

"her clothes are pretty . . . wore beige" [footnote]: Morrow, 2; quoted in Dolby, 40.

transparent umbrellas [footnote]: see Hughes, 25.

two hundred to three hundred letters: see Shawcross, *Queen and County*, 92.

"Barring cataclysm": Prochaska, 315.

"long drawn-out . . . in perspective": quoted in Smith, *Elizabeth the Queen*, 375.

"The best thing for her": quoted (with modern grammatical amendments) in Worsley, *Queen Victoria*, 259.

"now I wish to live": Ibid., 276.

Even toddlers experience: see Santi, 12.

"when our compassion circuits": Ibid., 18.

"I find this amazing": see "How to Make Stress Your Friend," a TED Talk by Kelly McGonigal, June 2013.

blood pressure, cholesterol . . . "Hand hygiene" [footnote]: see Santi, 22; A. M. Grant and D. A. Hofmann, "It's Not All about Me: Motivating Hand Hygiene among Health Care Professionals by Focusing on Patients," *Psychology Science* 22 (2011): 1494–1499; referenced in Strecher, 74.

"her awakening": quoted in Paxman, *On Royalty*, 231.

"to feel I am needed": quoted in Smith, *Diana in Search*, 190.

"support and love . . . carried me through": Ibid., 189.

"You don't think about yourself": quoted in Hamilton, 118.

"easier American . . . I joined up": quoted in Spoto, 246, 251.

"two sizes . . . only get worse" [footnote]: see "Princess Diana Detailed Her Memorable Meeting with Grace Kelly and Elizabeth Taylor" by Hilary Weaver, *Vanity Fair*, June 15, 2017.

Yale and Harvard researchers: C. Mogilner et al., "Giving Time Gives You Time," *Psychological Science* 23 (2012): 1233–1238.

"Giving time gives": Ibid.

"It sure explains how": Santi, 27.

640 engagements: see "Princess Anne, the Princess Royal: The Hardest Working Royal" by Rachel Martin, *Woman* magazine, September 1, 2017.

"Not bloody likely!": quoted in Smith, *Elizabeth the Queen*, 255.

"the exhilaration of others": quoted in "The Queen Mother in Her Own Words" compiled by Rajeev Syal and Sean Rayment, *Telegraph*, March 31, 2002.

"The point of human life": quoted in Smith, *Elizabeth the Queen*, 78.

In 2001, aged 100 . . . old and loyal servant: see Shawcross, *Counting One's Blessings*, 619.

"quite simply, it is the people": "The Queen Mother," *Telegraph*.

1950s, when scientists: see Santi, 20.

"We noticed that the most": quoted in Buettner, *The Blue Zones*, 190.

A five-year American study: M. Poulin et al., "Giving to Others and the Association between Stress and Mortality," *American Journal of Public Health* 103 (2013): 1649–1655.

recently totaling 780: see Seward, *My Husband and I*, 272.

"you can't play . . . All this is yours!" [footnote]: quoted in Eade, 49.

"kindness in another's": "Christmas Broadcast 1992," Royal Household website; royal.uk, December 25, 1992.

OFF WITH THEIR HEADS

You don't know that you are [opening quote]: Burnett, 157.

"If any person": quoted, using female pronouns, in Huish, 264.

By 1830, however: see Glenn, 77.

like the Royal Falconer: see *Penelope Keith: At Her Majesty's Service*, directed by Zoe Dobson, Chanel 4, June 5, 2016, episodes 1, 2.

Herb Strewer one Jessica Fellowes [footnote]: Ibid.

a chartered accountant: see "Did You Know the Queen Still Has a 'Champion'?" by Charlotte Mayhew, *Tatler*, August 8, 2019.

"I am tempted to suggest": quoted in Shawcross, *Queen and County*, 165.

"freeze out": Longford, 125.

"non-persons": see Brandreth, 73.

"the equivalent of being": Seward, *The Queen's Speech*, 199.

hapless Marion Crawford . . . death in 1988: see Tinniswood, 319–320.

"doing a Crawfie": see Longford, 128.

"intimate enough to address": Parker, 151.

"nice dull people . . . gold": quoted in Shawcross, *Counting One's Blessings*, 214.

"The Crown . . . lonely splendour": Tennyson, *The Works*, 433.

During the 1950s [footnote]: see Eade, 217.

"slightly mysterious Department": quoted in Hardman, *Queen of the World*, 10.

"she's the inventor": Claire Foy in discussion with Chelsea Handler in "The Crown's Claire Foy," *Chelsea*, Netflix, December 7, 2017.

"strength and stay": quoted in Shawcross, *Queen and Country*, 216.

"a bloody fool": quoted in Brandreth, 208.

"herself from the blistering": Erickson, *Lilibet*, 196.

S O U R C E N O T E S · 263

"I'm simply not going": Ibid., 196.

"kindness, sympathy": quoted in Greene, 49.

"emotional contagion": see Christakis, 35.

Queen Mary was a master: see Longford, 313.

"Oh, do shut up": quoted in Brandreth, 249.

"tolerance is the one": quoted in Dolby, 81.

"Carry on with your house party": quoted in Bradford, 405.

"as if they were small children": Robertson, 100.

Louis Mountbatten believed: see Bradford, 401.

"most people can hide": Ibid., 401.

"a united family": quoted in Shawcross, *Counting One's Blessings*, 216.

"That's the most pompous" [footnote]: quoted in Longford, 342.

"one can only wonder": quoted in King.

Edward was barred from his brother's: see Shawcross, *Queen and Country*, 142.

"What a smug stinking": quoted in "Letters to Duchess of Windsor: Duke
    Called Relatives 'Seedy Bunch of Old Hags,'" *Los Angeles Times*, June 20,
    1988.

"true aristocrats are perhaps": Lyall, 2, 117.

"the political perma-smile": quoted in Smith, *Elizabeth the Queen*, 470.

"at the heart of Britain's": Lacey, *Monarch*, 7.

"Exactly like petrol . . . offer her a drink" [footnote]: quoted in Brown, *Nine-
    ty-Nine Glimpses*, 14, 339.

"I am very glad to be": quoted in "Duty Is the Key to the Queen's Success" by
    Lucy Draper, *Newsweek*, June 19, 2015.

If she reads for pleasure: see "Jubilee Reading, Fit for a Queen" by David Barnett,
    Guardian, May 4, 2012; Dolby.

"be quiet": see "Miriam's Queen Fear," *Daily Express*, October 15, 2007.

"The trouble with behaving": quoted in Shawcross, *Queen and Country*, 163.

"kidnapped my sleep": Ferguson, *What I Know* Now, 22.

"You don't know what . . . became my friend": Ibid., 99.

"Great-Fun Fergie": Ibid., 21.

"[I] completely believed": quoted in Petrella, 119.

"You caused me . . . little to do with us" [footnote]: Ferguson, *What I Know Now*,
    21–22.

Oliver Cromwell . . . hanged: see "The Royal Soap Opera" by Malcolm Mugger-
    idge, *New Statesman*, 1955.

most likable member . . . 4 percent: see Smith, *Prince Charles*, 271–272.

"freedom in being disliked": Kishimi, 144.

"I wish I'd had the courage": see Ware, 37.

"The idea that you don't": quoted in Smith, *Elizabeth the Queen*, 236.

"The Queen, mummy": quoted in "50 Other Things You Didn't Know about the Queen" by Euan Ferguson, *Guardian*, January 26, 2002.

SOME ONE ELSE

More things are wrought by prayer [opening quote]: Tennyson, *Idylls of the King*, 416.

"Godless Florin" [footnote]: see Seward, *My Husband and I*, 261.

"this blessed plot": Shakespeare, *Richard II*, 33.

"people see the monarchy": Longford, 346.

England lasted little more: see Paxman, *On Royalty*, introduction.

"Some One Else was": Ibid., 126.

"It seemed that these": Ibid., 126.

Post-coronation Britain: see Shawcross, *Queen and County*, 73.

"God's representative in this realm": quoted in Brown, *Ninety-Nine Glimpses*, 293; Bradley, xvi.

"is the absolute mainspring": Ibid., 195.

"The Queen is a person": quoted in Seward, *My Husband and I*, 94.

She attends church . . . in prayer: see Hoey, *We Are Amused*, 173; Seward, *My Husband and I*, 257–258; Brandreth, 290.

reading a chapter of the Bible: see Shawcross, *The Queen Mother*, 41.

"While she may guard": Greene, 32.

He is her self-avowed "inspiration . . . anchor": Ibid., 32.

"carelessly throw away": quoted in Shawcross, *Queen and Country*, 197.

"I know just how much": quoted in Greene, 6.

"external locus of control": see Buettner, *The Blue Zones*, 209–210.

"not what makes the engine": Ferguson, *What I Know Now*, 92.

It was Elizabeth's idea: see Greene, 9.

"And I said to the man": "God Knows" by Minnie Louise Haskins, quoted in Knowles, *Modern Quotations*, 147.

"Prince of Peace": see Greene, 43.

"She's got a capacity": quoted in Smith, *Elizabeth the Queen*, 264.

"Healthy centenarians . . . looking out for them": Buettner, *The Blue Zones*, 103, 209–210, 287.

"In 2009 one of the" [footnote]: M. E. McCullough and B. L. B. Willoughby, "Religion, Self-Regulation, and Self-Control: Associations, Explanations, and Implications," *Psychological Bulletin* 135 (2009): 69–93; referenced in Baumeister, 179.

"Duke University . . . Stanford" [footnote]: H. G. Koenig et al., "Attendance at Religious Services, Interleukin-6, and Other Biological Indicators of Immune Function in Older Adults," *International Journal of Psychiatry in Medicine* 27 (1997): 233–250; referenced in Tolson, 53.

"to talk to Mummy": quoted in Junor, *Prince William*, 113.

"there is comfort to be had": Brandreth, 324.

She prefers the ancient . . . King James: see Bradford, 499; Hoey, *Life with the Queen*, 159.

never been dogmatic: see Brandreth, 290.

meet a Catholic pope: see Greene, 42.

"traditional and uncomplicated": Shawcross, *The Queen Mother*, 905.

"the Christian message": quoted in Shawcross, *Queen and Country*, 237.

"believing that if a preacher" [footnote]: Seward, *My Husband and I*, 266.

"the mind and soul" [footnote]: quoted in Hoey, *Life with the Queen*, 160.

"Go forth into the world": Ibid., 237.

Religion, as its root implies: see Ackroyd, 316.

"Religious conviction": quoted in Brandreth, 282.

"The long caravan . . . snake-oil salesman": Paxman, *On Royalty*, 140.

"as much a part of [her] daily": Seward, *My Husband and I*, 257–258.

"For Christians, as for all": quoted in Greene, 56.

"Whether in a church, a field": Lubomirski, 57.

her Diamond Jubilee: see "The Queen's Diamond Jubilee: Happy and Glorious, the River Queen" by Gordon Rayner, *Telegraph*, June 3, 2012.

"life was only the beginning": Ackroyd, 130.

"eternal recurrence" [footnote]: see Heidegger, 25.

corruptible crown for an incorruptible: paraphrasing the last words of Charles I, quoted in Hamilton, 25.

"she has her luggage packed": quoted in Shawcross, *Queen and Country*, 195.

AGE LIKE A QUEEN: OVERVIEW

May heaven, great monarch [opening quote]: Dryden, 197.

Be willing to be old [opening quote]: MacDonald, 51.

Her journal entry: see Rappaport, 118–119.

Unable to mount: Williams, *Young Elizabeth*, 299.

stood for nearly four hours: see "Diamond Jubilee 2012: Four Hours in the Freezing Rain at 86! How Did the Queen Do It?" by Robert Hardman, *Daily Mail*, June 3, 2012.

purpose-built "throne": see "The Queen's Diamond Jubilee: Happy and Glorious, the River Queen" by Gordon Rayner, *Telegraph*, June 3, 2012.

"Anyone can get old": quoted in Seward, *The Queen's Speech*, 196.

Roughly 75 percent more [footnote]: J. V. B. Hjelmborg et al., "Genetic Influence on Human Lifespan and Longevity," *Human Genetics* (2006): 312–321; referenced Buettner, *The Blue Zones*, xxii.

"the Queen wills it": see Smith, *English History Made Brief*, 19.

RADIANCE

To be stable in so public [opening quote]: Pope-Hennessy, 431.

I did not feel my best [opening quote]: Hamilton, 149.

"In place of a Dark Lord": *The Lord of the Rings: The Fellowship of the Ring*, directed by Peter Jackson (New York, NY: New Line Cinema, 2001).

"It makes her look like": quoted in Hoban, 137.

"Freud should be locked": quoted in "Freud Royal Portrait Divides Critics," BBC News, December 21, 2001.

"'before' half of a": see "Beneath the Skin of a Painted Lady: The Best Royal Portrait for 150 Years" by Adrian Searle, *Guardian*, December 21, 2001.

"a travesty": quoted in "Freud Royal Portrait," BBC News.

"the body politic": see Kantorowicz.

The medieval doctrine . . . "I am but one" [footnote]: see Waller, 3–4, 176.

"no longer [be]": quoted "Freud Royal Portrait," BBC News.

dressed either similarly or exactly: see Hughes, 174.

"to catch up": quoting Anne Glenconner in Smith, *Elizabeth the Queen*, 32.

"was immediately struck": quoted in Brandreth, 207.

"sugar pink" cheeks: quoted in Smith, *Elizabeth the Queen*, 32.

"I never realized . . . like that all over": Ibid., 48.

"luminous skin . . . beauty regimen": Ibid., 272, 433.

"The Queen's creamy": Morrow, 59.

Cyclax products on her face: Ibid., 59; Smith, *Elizabeth the Queen*, 273.

when it comes to makeup: see Smith, *Elizabeth the Queen*, 273.

"Balmoral" shade: see Andersen, *Game of Crowns*, 43.

professional makeup artist: see Kelly.

"Do you know she has" [footnote]: quoted in Shawcross, *The Queen Mother*, 235.

"movie star . . . Soap never" [footnote]: quoted in Spoto, 194.

"tightly permed white hair": Conrad, 73.

"I need to keep out": quoted in Smith, *Elizabeth the Queen*, 105.

"her skin leathered": "Princess Margaret's Beauty and Arrogance are On Parade in *Ninety-Nine Glimpses*" by Karen Heller, *Washington Post*, August 8, 2018.

puff through 60 in a day [footnote]: see "A Bad Habit She Found Hard to Kick" by David Harrison, *Telegraph*, February 10, 2002.

kippered . . . "not that close" [footnote]: see Brown, *Ninety-Nine Glimpses*, 15, 21, 165.

"weathering" activities: see Smith, *Elizabeth the Queen*, 272.

Snow White incarnate: see "An Elusive Icon: The Changing Face of Our Monarch" by Hannah Betts, *Telegraph*, February 7, 2012.

too rich or too thin: see Hamilton, 36.

"She wasn't slim and chic": Brandreth, 108.

"Fat Don't Crack": Harr, 116

"You'll have to lose" [footnote]: quoted in "Long May Prince Philip Continue to Speak His Mind" by Tom Utley, *Telegraph*, August 1, 2001.

"the BMI curve": quoted in "When Thinner Isn't Better" by Sandra Lamb, *AARP*, June 13, 2019.

"it turns out that": Claudia Kawas in discussion with Lesley Stahl, "*90+*" for *60 Minutes*, produced by Shari Finkelstein and Jennie Held, *CBS*, May 4, 2014.

artist Rolf Harris: see "Portrait Horribilis: Why It's So Hard to Draw the Queen" by Jonathan Jones, *Guardian*, April 12, 2016.

rarely looks at herself: see Hoey, *Life with the Queen*, 174.

"She [has] little patience": Smith, *Elizabeth the Queen*, 32.

hair done once a week . . . twice a day: Ibid., 469; Brown, *Ninety-Nine Glimpses*, 7.

"never cared a fig": Crawford, 29.

hint of cleavage . . . hemline: see Smith, *Elizabeth the Queen*, 32; Hoey, *Life with the Queen*, 108.

"to transform and transform": quoting Sam McKnight in Smith, *Diana in Search*, 17.

The nips and tucks: see Smith, *Elizabeth the Queen*, xiv.

"Windsor facelift . . . frank, unapologetic": "An Elusive Icon: The Changing Face of Our Monarch" by Hannah Betts, *Telegraph*, February 7, 2012.

"I would not like to feel": quoted in Petrella, 157.

268 · SOURCE NOTES

"Mask of Youth": see Weir, *The Life of Elizabeth I*, 239.

"Take kindly the counsel": Ehrmann.

"direct descendant . . . impossible to keep" quoted in "Queen Calls 1776 a Lesson That Aided Britain," *New York Times*, July 7, 1976.

JUBILEE ME

I am easier with myself [opening quote]: see Hamilton, 127.

"His Majesty's hope": quoted Williams, *Kind Regards*.

"centenarian team": see "Queen's 'Birthday Card Team' Expands to Cope with Surge of 100-Year-Olds" by John Bingham, *Telegraph*, September 25, 2014.

on her one-hundredth birthday [footnote]: see "A Birthday Greeting from Lilibet" by Stephen Bates, *Guardian*, August 4, 2000.

Botox injections: see "'Preventative Botox' Rising Trend Among Millennials" by Michelle Gant, *Fox News*, April 19, 2018.

"sans teeth, sans eyes": William Shakespeare quoted in Knowles, *Quotations*, 659.

"rage, rage against": Dylan Thomas quoted in Ibid., 772.

"got the giggles": Queen Mother quoted in Knowles, *Modern Quotations*, 104.

She veritably "blossomed": quoting Robert Salisbury in Smith, *Elizabeth the Queen*, 452.

"Never have I seen": quoting Annabel Goldsmith in Ibid., 453.

"[he] and I were in": Ibid., 453.

"Oh tell Malcolm": Ibid., 453.

"Things are much more fun": quoted in Erickson, *Lilibet*, 322.

"I am only just beginning": quoted in Shawcross, *Counting One's Blessings*, 191.

49 was the average: see "Mum's the Royal Word as Queen Mother Turns 100" by Marjorie Miller, *Los Angeles Times*, August 5, 2000.

"I always think of how": quoted in Shawcross, *Counting One's Blessings*, 574.

"The Private Secretary": quoted in Junor, *Prince Harry*, 161.

"became her best self": Worsley, *Queen Victoria*, 2.

"Britain as a whole": "Why Do We Still Have a Monarchy?" a lecture presented by Jeremy Paxman, King's College London, June 27, 2008.

"U-bend of life" . . . South America and Asia: see Greenstein, xiv, 10–12.

studies at Yale University: Ibid., 13, 187–188.

"radiated energy and robust": Erickson, *Lilibet*, 207.

"She has a theory": quoted in Smith, *Elizabeth the Queen*, 247.

"After all these years": quoted in Knowles, *Modern Quotations*, 104.

"It was wonderful to see": quoted in Shawcross, *The Queen Mother*, 926.

"ridiculous disease": quoted in Smith, *Elizabeth the Queen*, 246.

You were unwell that day: see Morgan, *The Audience*, 7.

"Such people at that time": Thompson, 127.

"as a dangerous drug . . . invariably worked!": Rhodes, 169.

"If you ignore illness": quoted in Hoey, *Life with the Queen*, 156.

a large study out of Norway [footnote]: L. I. Berge et. al., "Health Anxiety and Risk of Ischemic Heart Disease: A Prospective Cohort Study Linking the Hordaland Health Study (HUSK) with the Cardiovascular Diseases in Norway (CVDNOR) Project," *BMJ Open* (2016).

"She seemed indestructible": Hoey, *Life with the Queen*, 156.

"Get out! That's meant for Mummy!": quoted in Brown, *Ninety-Nine Glimpses*, 377.

"people who think" . . . Pessimistic grumps: Buettner, *The Blue Zones*, 183, 263.

"exceptional longevity": L. O. Lee et. al., "Optimism Is Associated with Exceptional Longevity in 2 Epidemiologic cohorts of men and women," *Proceedings of the National Academy of Sciences* 116 (2019): 18357–18362.

"I'm going to live to a hundred": quoted in Longford, 373.

main gist of homeopathy [footnote]: see Lockie, 10–13.

Her sinus infections . . . sore throats [footnote]: Smith, *Elizabeth the Queen*, 247; Shawcross, *The Queen Mother*, 553, 817.

developed a brain tumor [footnote]: Erickson, *Lilibet*, 207.

"effervescent enthusiasm for life": quoted in Shawcross, *Counting One's Blessings*, 568.

vibrant shades like daffodil yellow: see Hoey, *Life with the Queen*, 117.

"When you're young": Taylor, 52.

"warmer, more approachable": Smith, *Elizabeth the Queen*, 452.

"Twenty Four Reasons": see Brown, *Ninety-Nine Glimpses*, 270.

"I was born too late": quoted in Hoey, *Life with the Queen*, 149.

"growing more and more temperamental": Erickson, *Lilibet*, 223.

"Count your blessings!" Shawcross, *Counting One's Blessings*, 574.

how "heavenly" it was: Ibid., 621.

"She turned even the most . . . spending an afternoon": Rhodes, 162.

"Life ain't all you want": see Hampton, 121.

"tomorrow you might be": quoted in Shawcross, *Counting One's Blessings*, 619.

"She was so depressed" [footnote]: quoted in Taylor, 25.

THE MARMITE THEORY

Happiness . . . is neither [opening quote]: Yeats, 121.

refer to Elizabeth as "Gentlemen": see Smith, *Elizabeth the Queen*, 6.

"good things" and "bad things": see Sellar.

one of its greatest secrets of survival: see Williams, *Young Elizabeth*.

"the Marmite theory": quoting Robin Janvrin, Smith, *Elizabeth the Queen*, 419.

"the monarchy needed to change": Ibid., 419.

Queens didn't smile too frequently: see Shawcross, *Queen and Country*, 21.

"a priggish schoolgirl . . . loyal and constructive": "The Monarch Today," *National and English Review*, August 1957, 61–67.

"I felt it was . . . Empire Loyalists!" [footnote]: quoted in "Take That M'Lord!" *LIFE Magazine*, August 19, 1957, 38.

futuristic as the moon landing: see Hardman, *Her Majesty*.

elite pageantry of the Season: see Marr, 155.

Her cut-glass accent: Ibid., 312.

"the Queen has seen a staggering": Ibid., 311.

history's two famous Georges: see Bradford, 527.

US presidency . . . "We elect a king" [footnote]: see Paxman, *On Royalty*, 313; "A Point of View: Is the US President an Elected Monarch" by David Cannadine, BBC News, May 15, 2015.

"Yet bizarrely": Marr, 311.

"Change has become a constant": Ibid., 289.

"a private war with the twentieth": quoted in Pope-Hennessy, 551.

His "hatred of change": Bradford, 12–13.

fuss over the de-wigging . . . intercom: Erickson, *Lilibet*, 194.

"accelerating pace": quoted in Marr, 289.

rigidly "hardwired" [footnote]: see Diaz, 184; Levitin, 73.

George Dawson, aged 98 [footnote]: Dawson.

"unless I get Alzheimer's": quoted in Smith, *Elizabeth the Queen*, 515.

shaking hands with an oak tree: see Connolly, 123.

"as sharp as a needle": quoted in Shawcross, *Counting One's Blessings*, 76.

Queen Mary never enjoyed "resting" . . . "improving her mind": Pope-Hennessy, 434.

She watches television sparingly: see Hoey, *We Are Amused*, 126.

two crosswords . . . cheating: see Smith, *Elizabeth the Queen*, 70; Hoey, *Life with the Queen*, 91.

emergency puzzles in her handbag: see Andersen, *Game of Crowns*, 43.

an impressive four minutes: see Erickson, *Lilibet*, 316.

Sometimes stretching to 10,000 pieces: see Burgess, 161.

"impossible . . . about twenty pieces": Paxman, *On Royalty*, 4.

the Queen has been observed: see Bradford, 323.

problem-solving exercises . . . "among the most important" [footnote]: see Levitin, 132; Csikszentmihalyi, 121.

she trained with the Auxiliary: see Smith, *Elizabeth the Queen*, 21.

carburetor with her eyes closed: see Hoey, *Life with the Queen*, 6.

"a compartmentalized brain": quoted in Smith, *Elizabeth the Queen*, 168.

speaking in riddles: "Queen Elizabeth likes to 'Speak in Riddles,' has 'Nicknames for Everyone,' Claims Royal Expert" by Stephanie Nolasco, *Fox News*, March 9, 2019.

"Why does one have wax": Hamilton, 88.

"countryside woman of limited": quoted in Hardman, *Queen of the World*, 14.

"an extraordinarily shrewd": quoted in Shawcross, *Queen and Country*, 216.

"have gotten a first-class": Ibid., 11.

"overwhelmed by the occasion . . . Yes, Ma'am": quoted in Shawcross, *Queen and County*, 162.

LONDON BRIDGE

In my end is my beginning [opening quote]: see Knowles, *Modern Quotations*, 100.

BBC's quick response: see Burgess, 114.

M4 motorway . . . "royal [is] about to": see "London Bridge Is Down: The Secret Plan for the Days After the Queen's Death" by Sam Knight, *Guardian*, March 17, 2017.

she died incredibly peacefully [footnote]: see Smith, *Elizabeth the Queen*, 436; "Queen Mother Dies Peacefully, Aged 101," *Guardian*, March 30, 2002.

Prince Philip was postulated: see "The British Media Rehearses the Queen's Death at Least Once a Year" by Corinne Purtill, *pri.org*, April 21, 2016.

since the 1960s . . . "the next great rupture": "London Bridge," *Guardian*; Andersen, *Game of Crowns*, 12.

Many in the press rehearse: see Andersen, *Game of Crowns*, 13.

The Times reportedly . . . planned for 22 years: see "London Bridge," *Guardian*.

"I am always altering": quoted in Brown, *Ninety-Nine Glimpses*, 398.

Queen Victoria chose . . . "Operation Hope Not": see "London Bridge," *Guardian*.

"Tay Bridge . . . London Bridge": see Andersen, *Game of Crowns*, 12; Smith, *Elizabeth the Queen*, 397.

Downright "beastly": Shawcross, *Counting One's Blessings*, 511.

over half of all American adults: see "Survey: 60% Lack Will or Estate Planning" by Barbranda Lumpkins Walls, *AARP*, February 24, 2017.

"What a Waste!": Lady Colin Campbell in discussion with Andrew Morton and Anne Sebba, *Royal Wives at War*, directed by Tim Dunn, BBC Two, September 18, 2016.

"All my possessions for": quoted in Knowles, *Quotations*, 455.

"What a wonderful life": quoted in Rubin, *The Happiness Project*, 2.

"healthy and important": quoted in Smith, *Prince Charles*, 484.

"to take the long view": quoted in Greene, 6.

"held in trust" [footnote]: see Longford, 7.

"even on the most exalted": Montaigne, 317; quoted in Paxman, *On Royalty*, 25.

"So teach us to number": Psalm 90:12, *Holy Bible*, King James Version.

"of all mindfulness meditations": quoted in Rubin, *The Happiness Project*, 196.

mono no aware: see Davies, 37.

"remember that you will die": see Strecher, 97.

portrait of Elizabeth I: see Russell.

premeditatio malorum: see Pigliucci, 151.

"Let us prepare our minds": Seneca, *Moral Letters*, quoted in Holiday, *The Daily Stoic*, 357.

"were going to live ten thousand": quoted in Strecher, 94.

"autobiographical reasoning" [footnote]: see "Story of My Life: How Narrative Creates Personality" by Julie Beck, *Atlantic*, August 10, 2015.

"Always live your life" [footnote]: Pessl, 48.

"with the end in mind . . . your life as a whole": Covey, 105.

The Tombstone Test: see Strecher, 43, 57.

"If this were the last day": Winfrey, 13.

"All shall be well . . . her personal philosophy": Longford, 95, 316.

"On the dais stood the Queen": quoted in "A Life of Legend, Duty and Devotion" by John Ezard, *Guardian*, March 31, 2002.

At the thanksgiving service: Longford, 316.

"Mother Courage": "Mother Courage," *The Sydney Morning Herald*, April 1, 2002.

"The true measure of all": quoted in Seward, *The Queen's Speech*, 249.

with two bodies: see Waller, 4.

"The King is dead, long live": see Hoey, *We Are Amused*, 38.

the Royal Standard . . . "insensitive" [footnote]: Ibid.; "Diana: Let the Flag Fly at Half Mast" by Geoffrey Levy and Richard Kay, *Daily Mail*, September 4, 1997.

imagery of the phoenix: Paxman, *On Royalty*, 62.

"immortality project": Becker.

thinking in terms of "if only": quoted in Seward, *The Queen's Speech*, 161.

"God save Queen Elizabeth": DK, *Queen Elizabeth II*, 141.

Bibliography

Ackroyd, Peter. *Albion: The Origins of the English Imagination*. New York: Doubleday, 2003.

Airlie, Mabell, Countess of. *Thatched with Gold: The Memoirs*. Edited by Jennifer Ellis. London: Hutchinson, 1962.

Andersen, Christopher. *Game of Crowns: Elizabeth, Camilla, Kate, and the Throne*. New York: Gallery Books, 2016.

——. *William and Kate: A Royal Love Story*. New York: Simon and Schuster, 2011.

Princess Anne the Princess Royal, with Ivor Herbert. *Riding Through My Life*. London: Pelham, 1991.

Arbiter, Dickie. *On Duty With the Queen*. Dorking, UK: Blink Publishing, 2014.

Ashford, Brenda. *A Spoonful of Sugar: A Nanny's Story*. New York: Doubleday, 2013.

Aurelius, Marcus. *Meditations*. Translated by Maxwell Staniforth. London: Penguin Books, 1964.

Bagehot, Walter. *The English Constitution*. 1867. Reprint, London: Henry S. King, 1872.

Baumeister, Roy F., and John Tierney. *Willpower: Rediscovering the Greatest Human Strength*. New York: Penguin, 2011.

Becker, Ernest. *The Denial of Death*. New York: Free Press, 1973.

Bennett, Alan. *The Uncommon Reader*. New York: Farrar, Straus and Giroux, 2007.

Blair, Tony. *A Journey: My Political Life*. New York: Vintage Books, 2011.

Bradford, Sarah. *Elizabeth: A Biography of Britain's Queen*. New York: Farrar, Straus and Giroux, 1996.

Bradley, Ian. *God Save the Queen: The Spiritual Heart of the Monarchy*. London: Continuum, 2012.

Brandreth, Gyles. *Philip and Elizabeth: Portrait of a Royal Marriage*. New York: Norton, 2005.

Brannen, Barbara. *The Gift of Play: Why Adult Women Stop Playing and How to Start Again*. San Jose, CA: Writers Club Press, 2002.

Brones, Anna, and Joanna Kindvall. *Fika: The Art of the Swedish Coffee Break*. Berkeley, CA: Ten Speed Press, 2015.

Brown, Craig. *Ninety-Nine Glimpses of Princess Margaret*. New York: Farrar, Straus and Giroux, 2017.

Brown, Stuart, and Christopher Vaughan. *Play: How It Shapes the Brain, Opens the Imagination, and Invigorates the Soul*. New York: Avery, 2009.

Brown, Tina. *The Diana Chronicles*. New York: Doubleday, 2007.

Brown, Mike, and Carol Harris and C. J. Jackson. *The Ration Book Diet*. Stroud, UK: Sutton, 2004.

Buettner, Dan. *The Blue Zones: 9 Lessons for Living Longer from the People Who've Lived the Longest*. Washington, DC: National Geographic, 2012.

———. *The Blue Zones Solution: Eating and Living Like the World's Healthiest People*. Washington, DC: National Geographic, 2015.

Burgess, Colin. *Behind Palace Doors: My Service as the Queen Mother's Equerry*. London: John Blake, 2006.

Burnett, Frances Hodgson. *A Little Princess*. 1905; New York: Grosset and Dunlap, 1989.

Cain, Susan. *Quiet: The Power of Introverts in a World That Can't Stop Talking*. New York: Crown Publishing, 2013.

Carroll, Lewis. *Alice's Adventures in Wonderland* and *Through the Looking Glass*. 1872. Reprint, London: Penguin Books, 1998.

Casson, Sir Hugh, and Joyce Grenfell. *Nanny Says*. Edited by Diana, Lady Avebury. London: Dobson Books, 1972.

Chesterton, G. K. *The Collected Works of G. K. Chesterton*. Vol. 1, *Heretics, Orthodoxy, the Blatchford Controversies*, edited by David Dooley. San Francisco: Ignatius Press, 1986.

———. *G. K. Chesterton: The Dover Reader*. Mineola, NY: Dover Publications, 2014.

Churchill, Winston. *The Gathering Storm*. 1948; New York: Houghton Mifflin, 1976.

Christakis, Nicholas A., and James H. Fowler. *Connected: The Surprising Power of Our Social Networks and How They Shape Our Lives*. New York: Little, Brown, 2009.

Connolly, Tristanne, and Steve Clark, eds. *Liberating Medicine, 1720–1835*. London: Routledge, 2016.

Conrad, Peter. *Mythomania: Tales of Our Times, From Apple to ISIS*. New York: Thames and Hudson, 2016.

Covey, Stephen R. *The 7 Habits of Highly Effective People*. New York: Simon and Schuster, 1989.

Crawford, Marion. *The Little Princesses*. New York: Harcourt, 1950.

Crossman, Richard. *The Diaries of a Cabinet Minister*. Vol. 2, *Lord President of the Council and Leader of the House of Commons, 1966–68*. London: Jonathan Cape, 1976.

Csikszentmihalyi, Mihaly. *Flow: The Psychology of Optimal Experience.* New York: Harper Perennial, 2008.

Dahl, Roald. *The BFG.* 1982; New York: Puffin, 2013.

Davies, Rojer J, and Osamu Ikeno. *The Japanese Mind: Understanding Contemporary Japanese Culture.* North Clarendon, VT: Tuttle Publishing, 2011.

Dawson, George, and Richard Glaubman. *Life Is So Good.* New York: Random House, 2000.

Day, David. *An Encyclopedia of Tolkien: The History and Mythology That Inspired Tolkien's World.* San Diego, CA: Canterbury Classics, 2019.

Diaz, Cameron, with Sandra Bark. *The Longevity Book: The Science of Aging, the Biology of Strength, and the Privilege of Time.* New York: HarperCollins, 2016.

Dimbleby, Jonathan. *The Prince of Wales: A Biography.* New York: W. Morrow, 1994.

Dixon, Thomas. *Weeping Britannia: Portrait of a Nation in Tears.* Oxford, UK: Oxford University Press, 2015.

DK, *Queen Elizabeth II and the Royal Family.* New York: Penguin Random House, 2015.

Dolby, Karen. *The Wicked Wit of Queen Elizabeth II.* New York: Berkley, 2017.

Dryden, John, and Sir Walter Scott. *The Works of John Dryden.* Vol. 5, *Amboyna; The State of Innocence; Aureng-Zebe; All for Love.* London: William Miller, 1808.

Duhigg, Charles. *The Power of Habit. Why We Do What We Do in Life and Business.* New York: Random House, 2012.

Dunne, Claire. *Carl Jung: Wounded Healer of the Soul.* London: Watkins, 2015.

Eade, Philip. *Prince Philip: The Turbulent Early Life of the Man Who Married Queen Elizabeth II.* New York: Henry Holt, 2011.

Edwards, Anne. *Matriarch: Queen Mary and the House of Windsor.* 1984; Lanham, MD: Rowman and Littlefield, 2015.

Ehrmann, Max. *Desiderata: Words for Life.* New York: Scholastic Press, 2003.

Erickson, Carolly. *Lilibet: An Intimate Portrait of Elizabeth II.* Waterville, ME: Thorndike Press, 2004.

———. *Royal Panoply: Brief Lives of the English Monarchs.* New York: St. Martin's Press, 2006.

Fellowes, Jessica. *The Wit and Wisdom of Downton Abbey.* New York: St. Martin's Griffin, 2015.

Ferguson, Sarah. *Finding Sarah: A Duchess's Journey to Find Herself.* New York: Atria Books, 2011.

———. *What I Know Now: Simple Lessons Learned the Hard Way.* New York: Simon and Schuster, 2003.

Flanagan, Mark, and Edward Griffiths. *A Royal Cookbook: Seasonal Recipes from Buckingham Palace.* London: Royal Collection Trust, 2014.

Fleming, Ian. *On Her Majesty's Secret Service.* New York: Signet Books, 1963.

Forbes, Grania. *My Darling Buffy: The Early Life of the Queen Mother.* London: Headline, 1999.

Fox, Kate. *Watching the English: The Hidden Rules of English Behavior.* London: Hodder and Stoughton, 2014.

Frankl, Viktor. *Man's Search for Meaning.* 1946; Boston: Beacon Press, 1992.

Fredrickson, Barbara L. *Positivity.* New York: Crown Publishers, 2009.

Friedman, Howard S., and Leslie R. Martin. *The Longevity Project: Surprising Discoveries for Health and Long Life from the Landmark Eight-Decade Study.* New York: Hudson Stress Press, 2011.

Furedi, Frank. *Therapy Culture: Cultivating Vulnerability in an Uncertain Age.* London: Routledge, 2004.

Garcia, Hector, and Francesc Miralles. *Ikigai: The Japanese Secret to a Long and Happy Life.* New York: Penguin Books, 2017.

Gilbert, Elizabeth. *Eat, Pray, Love: A Woman's Search for Everything Across Italy, India, and Indonesia.* New York: Penguin, 2006.

Glenn, Justin. *The Washingtons: A Family History.* Vol. 3, *Royal Descendants of the Presidential Branch.* El Dorado Hills, CA: Savas Publishing, 2015.

Gordon, Peter, and Denis Lawton. *Royal Education: Past, Present and Future.* London: Frank Cass, 1999.

Greene, Mark, and Catherine Butcher. *The Servant Queen and the King She Serves.* Swindon, UK: Bible Society, 2016.

Greenstein, Mindy, and Jimmie Holland. *Lighter as We Go: Virtues, Character Strengths, and Aging.* Oxford: Oxford University Press, 2015.

Hadot, Pierre. *Philosophy as a Way of Life: Spiritual Exercises from Socrates to Foucault.* Translated by Michael Chase. Malden, MA: Blackwell, 1995.

Hamilton, Alan. *We Are Amused: Over 500 Years of Bon Mots By and About the Royal Family.* London: Robert Hale, 2003.

Hampton, Janie. *How the Girl Guides Won the War.* London: Harper Press, 2010.

Hardman, Robert. *Her Majesty: Queen Elizabeth II and Her Court.* New York: Pegasus Books, 2012.

———. *Queen of the World.* New York: Pegasus Books, 2019.

Hart, Miranda. *Is It Just Me?* London: Hodder and Stoughton, 2012.

Hayes, Tim. *Riding Home: The Power of Horses to Heal.* New York: St. Martin's Press, 2015.

Heidegger, Martin. *Nietzsche.* Vol. 2, *The Eternal Recurrence of the Same.* Translated by David Farrell Krell. New York: Harper and Row, 1984.

Heschel, Abraham. *The Sabbath: Its Meaning for Modern Man.* New York: Farrar, Straus and Giroux, 1977.

Hoban, Phoebe. *Lucian Freud: Eyes Wide Open.* New York: Houghton Mifflin Harcourt, 2014.

Hoey, Brian. *Life with the Queen.* Stroud, UK: Sutton, 2006.

———. *Not in Front of the Corgis: Secrets of Life Behind the Royal Curtains.* London: Robson Press, 2011.

———. *We Are Amused: A Royal Miscellany.* London: JR Books, 2010.

Holden, Katherine. *Nanny Knows Best: The History of the British Nanny, from Mary Poppins to Supernanny.* Stroud, UK: The History Press, 2013.

Holiday, Ryan. *The Obstacle Is the Way: The Timeless Art of Turning Trials into Triumph.* New York: Portfolio/Penguin, 2014.

Holiday, Ryan, and Stephen Hanselman. *The Daily Stoic: 366 Meditations on Wisdom, Perseverance, and the Art of Living.* New York: Penguin, 2016.

Hughes, Sali. *Our Rainbow Queen: A Tribute to Queen Elizabeth II and Her Colorful Wardrobe.* New York: Plume/Penguin, 2019.

Huish, Robert. *An Authentic History of the Coronation of His Majesty George IV.* London: J. Robins and Co. Albion Press, 1821.

Ingrams, Richard, ed. *England: An Anthology.* London: Collins, 1989.

Irvine, William B. *A Guide to the Good Life: The Ancient Art of Stoic Joy.* Oxford: Oxford University Press, 2009.

Jaques, Susan. *The Caesar of Paris: Napoleon Bonaparte, Rome, and the Artistic Obsession that Shaped an Empire.* New York: Pegasus Books, 2018.

Junor, Penny. *Prince Harry: Brother, Soldier, Son.* New York: Grand Central Publishing, 2014.

———. *Prince William: The Man Who Will Be King.* New York: Pegasus Books, 2014.

Kantorowicz, Ernst H. *The King's Two Bodies: A Study in Medieval Political Theology.* Princeton, NJ: Princeton University Press, 2016.

Kaplan, Rachel, and Stephen Kaplan. *The Experience of Nature: A Psychological Perspective.* New York: Cambridge University Press, 1989.

Keller, Gary, and Jay Papasan. *The One Thing: The Surprising Simple Truth Behind Extraordinary Results.* Austin, TX: Bard Press, 2012.

Kelly, Angela. *The Other Side of the Coin: The Queen, the Dresser and the Wardrobe.* London: HarperCollins, 2019.

King, Greg. *The Duchess of Windsor: The Uncommon Life of Wallis Simpson.* New York: Citadel Press, 1999.

Kishimi, Ichiro, and Fumitake Koga. *The Courage to Be Disliked: The Japanese Phenomenon that Shows You How to Change Your Life and Achieve Real Happiness.* New York: Atria Books, 2018.

Knowles, Elizabeth, ed. *The Oxford Dictionary of Quotations.* 5th ed. Oxford: Oxford University Press, 1999.

———. *The Oxford Dictionary of Modern Quotations*, 3rd ed. Oxford: Oxford University Press, 2007.

Lacey, Robert. *Majesty.* New York: Harcourt Brace Jovanovich, 1977.

———. *The Crown: The Official Companion.* Vol. 1, *Elizabeth II, Winston Churchill, and the Making of a Young Queen (1947–1955).* New York: Crown Archetype, 2017.

———. *Monarch: The Life and Reign of Elizabeth II.* New York: Free Press, 2002.

Lear, Linda. *Beatrix Potter: A Life in Nature.* New York: St. Martin's Griffin, 2007.

Lee, Laurie. *The Illustrated Cider with Rosie.* 1959; London: Cresset Press, 1989.

Leibovitz, Annie. *Annie Leibovitz At Work.* New York: Random House, 2008.

Levin, Carole. *The Reign of Elizabeth I.* New York: Palgrave, 2002.

Levine, James A. *Get Up! Why Your Chair Is Killing You and What You Can Do About It.* New York: St. Martin's Press, 2014.

Levine, Robert. *A Geography of Time: The Temporal Misadventures of a Social Psychologist, or How Every Culture Keeps Time Just a Little Bit Differently.* New York: Basic Books, 1997.

Levitin, David J. *Successful Aging: A Neuroscientist Explores the Power and Potential of Our Lives.* New York: Penguin, 2020.

Lewis, David. *Impulse: Why We Do What We Do Without Knowing Why We Do It.* Cambridge, MA: Harvard University Press, 2013.

Li, Qing. *Forest Bathing: How Trees Can Help You Find Health and Happiness.* New York: Viking, 2018.

Lockie, Andrew, and Nicola Geddes. *The Complete Guide to Homeopathy.* London: D. Kindersley, 1995.

Logue, Alexandra W. *The Psychology of Eating and Drinking*, 4th ed. New York: Routledge, 2015.

Longford, Elizabeth. *The Queen: The Life of Elizabeth II.* New York: Knopf, 1983.

Longmate, Norman. *How We Lived Then: A History of Everyday Life during the Second World War.* London: Hutchinson, 1971.

Lubbock, John. *The Use of Life.* London: Macmillan, 1895.

Lubomirski, Alexi. *Princely Advice for a Happy Life.* Kansas City: Andrews McMeel Publishing, 2015.

Lukianoff, Greg, and Jonathan Haidt. *The Coddling of the American Mind: How Good Intentions and Bad Ideas Are Setting Up a Generation for Failure.* New York: Penguin Press, 2018.

Lyall, Sarah. *The Anglo Files: A Field Guide to the British.* New York: W. W. Norton, 2008.

MacDonald, George. *The Poetical Works of George MacDonald.* Vol. 1. London: Chatto and Windus, 1893.

Mandler, Peter. *The English National Character: The History of an Idea from Edmund Burke to Tony Blair.* New Haven, CT: Yale University Press, 2006.

Marino, Gordon, ed. *The Quotable Kierkegaard.* Princeton, NJ: Princeton University Press, 2014.

Marr, Andrew. *The Real Elizabeth: An Intimate Portrait of Queen Elizabeth II.* New York: Henry Holt, 2012.

Mirren, Helen. *In the Frame: My Life in Words and Pictures.* New York: Atria Books, 2008.

Mischel, Walter. *The Marshmallow Test: Mastering Self-Control.* New York: Little, Brown, 2014.

Montaigne, Michel de. *The Essays of Michel de Montaigne.* Translated by Jacob Zeitlin. New York: Knopf, 1936.

Morgan, John. *Debrett's New Guide to Etiquette & Modern Manners: The Indispensable Handbook.* New York: St. Martin's Press, 2001.

Morgan, Peter. *The Audience.* New York: Dramatists Play Services, 2013.

Morrow, Ann. *The Queen.* New York: W. Morrow, 1983.

Morton, Andrew. *Diana: Her True Story—In Her Own Words.* 1992; New York: Simon and Schuster, 2017.

———. *Wallis in Love: The Untold Life of the Duchess of Windsor, the Woman Who Changed the Monarchy.* New York: Grand Central Publishing, 2018.

Murdoch, Iris. *The Nice and the Good.* 1968; London: Triad/Panther, 1977.

———. *The Sea, The Sea.* 1978; London: Vintage Books, 1999.

Oliver, Charles. *Dinner at Buckingham Palace.* Edited by Richard Warwick. Englewood Cliffs, NJ: Prentice-Hall, 1972.

Pang, Alex Soojung-Kim. *Rest: Why You Get More Done When You Work Less.* New York: Basic Books, 2016.

Paterson, Michael. *A Brief History of the Private Life of Elizabeth II.* New York: Little, Brown, 2012.

———. *Winston Churchill: Personal Accounts of the Great Leader at War.* Newton Abbot, UK: David and Charles, 2005.

Parker, Eileen. *Step Aside for Royalty: A Personal Experience.* London: Bachman and Turner, 1982.

Paxman, Jeremy. *On Royalty: A Very Polite Inquiry into Some Strangely Related Families.* New York: PublicAffairs, 2007.

———. *The English: A Portrait of a People.* Woodstock, NY: Overlook Press, 2000.

Pessl, Marisha. *Special Topics in Calamity Physics.* New York: Viking, 2006.

Peterson, Jordan. *12 Rules for Life: An Antidote to Chaos.* Toronto: Random House Canada, 2018.

Petrella, Kate. *Royal Wisdom: The Most Daft, Cheeky, and Brilliant Quotes from Britain's Royal Family.* Avon, MA: Adams Media, 2011.

Pierlot, Holly. *A Mother's Rule of Life: How to Bring Order to Your Home and Peace to Your Soul.* Manchester, NH: Sophia Institute Press, 2004.

Pigliucci, Massimo. *How to Be a Stoic: Using Ancient Philosophy to Live a Modern Life.* New York: Basic Books, 2017.

Pimlott, Ben. *The Queen: Elizabeth II and the Monarchy.* New York: HarperCollins, 2001.

Plato. *The Republic.* Harmondsworth, UK: Penguin, 1955.

Pope, Alexander. *Translation of the Iliad of Homer.* Hartford, UK: Silas Andrus and Son, 1851.

Pope-Hennessy, James. *Queen Mary.* 1959; London: Phoenix Press, 2000.

Porter, Kathleen. *Healthy Posture for Babies and Children: Tools for Helping Children to Sit, Stand, and Walk Naturally.* New York: Simon and Schuster, 2017.

Price, Catherine. *How to Break Up with Your Phone.* New York: Ten Speed Press, 2019.

Prochaska, Frank. *Royal Bounty: The Making of a Welfare Monarchy.* New Haven, CT: Yale University Press, 1995.

Rappaport, Helen. *Queen Victoria: A Biographical Companion.* Santa Barbara, CA: ABC-CLIO, 2003.

Ratcliff, Edward C, ed. *The Coronation Service of Her Majesty Queen Elizabeth II.* Cambridge, UK: Cambridge University Press, 1953.

Reagan, Ronald. *The Reagan Diaries.* New York: HarperCollins, 2009.

Rhodes, Margaret. *The Final Curtsey: A Royal Memoir by the Queen's Cousin.* Edinburgh: Birlinn, 2012.

Robertson, Donald. *Stoicism and the Art of Happiness: Practical Wisdom for Everyday Life.* London: John Murray Learning, 2018.

Rubin, Gretchen. *Better than Before: Mastering the Habits of Our Everyday Lives.* New York: Crown Publishers, 2015.

———. *The Happiness Project.* New York: HarperCollins, 2018.

Russell, Gareth. *An Illustrated Introduction to the Tudors.* Stroud, UK: Amberley Publishing, 2014.

Salmon, Hugh. *Thoughts on Life and Advertising.* Kibworth, UK: Troubador Publishing, 2018.

Santi, Jenny. *The Giving Way to Happiness: Stories and Science Behind the Life-Changing Power of Giving.* New York: Penguin Random House, 2015.

Scruton, Roger. *England: An Elegy.* London: Continuum, 2006.

Sebba, Anna. *That Woman: The Life of Wallis Simpson, Duchess of Windsor.* New York: St. Martin's Press, 2012.

Segar, Michelle. *No Sweat: How the Simple Science of Motivation Can Bring You a Lifetime of Fitness.* New York: AMACOM, 2015.

Seneca. *Moral and Political Essays.* Edited by John M. Cooper and J. F. Procopé. Cambridge, UK: Cambridge University Press, 1995.

Sellar, W. C., and R. J. Yeatman. *1066 and All That: A Memorable History of England.* London: Metheun Publishing, 1930.

Seward, Ingrid. *My Husband and I: The Inside Story of 70 Years of the Royal Marriage.* London: Simon and Schuster UK, 2017.

———. *The Queen's Speech: An Intimate Portrait of the Queen in Her Own Words.* London: Simon and Schuster, 2015.

Shakespeare, William. *Henry VI.* New Haven, CT: Yale University Press, 1923.

———. *Richard II.* New Haven, CT: Yale University Press, 1957.

Shawcross, William. *Counting One's Blessings: The Selected Letters of Queen Elizabeth the Queen Mother.* New York: Farrar, Straus and Giroux, 2012.

———. *Queen and Country: The Fifty-Year Reign of Elizabeth II.* New York: Simon and Schuster, 2002.

———. *The Queen Mother: The Official Biography.* New York: Knopf, 2009.

Shinn, Florence Scovel. *The Wisdom of Florence Scovel Shinn.* New York: Simon and Schuster, 1989.

Sissons, Michael, and Philip French, eds. *Age of Austerity.* London: Hodder and Stoughton, 1963.

Smith, Amanda, ed. *Hostage to Fortune: The Letters of Joseph P. Kennedy.* New York: Penguin, 2002.

Smith, Lacey Baldwin. *English History Made Brief, Irreverent, and Pleasurable.* Chicago: Academy Chicago Publishers, 2007.

Smith, Sally Bedell. *Elizabeth the Queen: The Life of a Modern Monarch.* New York: Random House, 2012.

———. *Diana in Search of Herself: Portrait of a Troubled Princess.* New York: Times Books, 1999.

———. *Prince Charles: The Passions and Paradoxes of an Improbable Life.* New York: Random House, 2017.

Sommers, Christina Hoff, and Sally Satel. *One Nation Under Therapy: How the Helping Culture Is Eroding Self-Reliance.* New York: St. Martin's Press, 2005.

Spark, Muriel. *The Girls of Slender Means.* New York: Knopf, 1963.

Spoto, Donald. *High Society: The Life of Grace Kelly.* New York: Three Rivers Press, 2009.

Stalker, Nancy K., ed. *Devouring Japan: Global Perspectives on Japanese Culinary Identity*. New York: Oxford University Press, 2018.

Starkey, David. *Crown and Country: A History of England through the Monarchy*. London: HarperPress, 2010.

Starrett, Kelly, with Juliet Starrett and Glen Cordoza. *Deskbound: Standing Up to a Sitting World*. Las Vegas, NV: Victory Belt Publishing, 2016.

Strecher, Victor J. *Life on Purpose: How Living for What Matters Most Changes Everything*. New York: HarperOne, 2016.

Strong, Roy C., and Cecil Beaton. *Cecil Beaton: The Royal Portraits*. New York: Simon and Schuster, 1988.

Taylor, Elizabeth. *Elizabeth Takes Off: On Weight Gain, Weight Loss, Self-Image, and Self-Esteem*. New York: Berkley Books, 1987.

Tennyson, Alfred. *Idylls of the King*. 1859; London: Macmillan, 1908.

———. *The Works of Alfred Lord Tennyson*. Ware, UK: Wordsworth Editions, 1994.

Thompson, Flora. *Lark Rise to Candleford: A Trilogy*. 1939; Boston: David R. Godine, 2009.

Tinniswood, Adrian. *Behind the Throne: A Domestic History of the British Royal Household*. New York: Basic Books, 2018.

Tolkien, J. R. R. *The Return of the King*. 1955; Boston: Houghton Mifflin, 2002.

Tolson, Chester L., and Harold G. Koenig. *The Healing Power of Prayer: The Surprising Connection Between Prayer and Your Health*. Grand Rapids, MI: Baker Books, 2004.

Various. *The Queen: A Penguin Special*. London: Penguin, 1977.

Visser, Margaret. *The Rituals of Dinner: The Origins, Evolution, Eccentricities, and Meaning of Table Manners*. New York: Grove Weidenfeld, 1991.

Waller, Maureen. *Sovereign Ladies: The Six Reigning Queens of England*. New York: St. Martin's Press, 2006.

Wansink, Brian. *Mindless Eating: Why We Eat More Than We Think*. New York: Bantam Books, 2006.

Ware, Bronnie. *The Top Five Regrets of the Dying: A Life Transformed by the Dearly Departing*. London: Hay House, 2011.

Weir, Alison. *Henry VIII: The King and His Court*. New York: Ballantine Books, 2008.

———. *The Life of Elizabeth I*. 1998; New York: Ballantine Books, 2008.

White, T. H. *The Book of Merlyn: The Unpublished Conclusion to "The Once and Future King."* Austin, TX: University of Texas Press, 2012.

Williams, Kate. *Young Elizabeth: The Making of the Queen*. New York: Pegasus Books, 2015.

Williams, Liz. *Kind Regards: The Lost Art of Letter Writing.* London: Michael O'Mara Books, 2012.

Winfrey, Oprah. *What I Know for Sure.* New York: Flatiron Books, 2014.

Worsley, Lucy, in association with Historic Royal Palaces. *Chocolate Fit for a Queen.* London: Edbury Press, 2015.

———. *Queen Victoria: Twenty-Four Days that Changed Her Life.* New York: St. Martin's Press, 2019.

Yeats, John Butler. *J. B. Yeats Letters to His Son W. B. Yeats and Others, 1869–1922.* Edited by Joseph Hone. New York: E. P. Dutton, 1946.

York, Sarah, Duchess of. *Dieting with the Duchess: Secrets and Sensible Advice for a Great Body.* New York: Simon and Schuster, 1998.

About the Author

B RYAN K OZLOWSKI is a lifestyle and British culture researcher. Author of *The Jane Austen Diet,* along with three previous books, his works have appeared in *Vogue,* the *New York Times* and the *Washington Post.*

CPSIA information can be obtained
at www.ICGtesting.com
Printed in the USA
JSHW051603211020
8954JS00003B/44